D0494886

TALES FROM A
COUNTRY PRACTICE

TALES FROM A COUNTRY PRACTICE

Arthur Jackson

The
Leisure
Circle

Copyright © 1986 by Souvenir Press Ltd

First published 1986 by Souvenir Press Ltd

This edition specially produced for
The Leisure Circle Limited by
Souvenir Press Ltd., 43 Great Russell Street,
London WC1B 3PA

All Rights Reserved. No part of this publication
may be reproduced, stored in a retrieval system,
or transmitted, in any form or by any means, electronic,
mechanical, photocopying, recording or otherwise without
the prior permission of the Copyright owner

ISBN 0 285 62740 6

Photoset and printed in Great Britain by
Redwood Burn Limited
Trowbridge, Wiltshire

Any tapestry of experience must be woven with the threads of imagination. While the house and events described in this book are based on fact, the characters are composites of many people I have met along the way, not necessarily in the context in which they appear.

The medical events described are the bread and butter of general practice; they happen to someone, somewhere, every day.

If any of my friends – or patients – think that they recognise themselves or each other, I am flattered, but they are mistaken. The only people who appear as they really are in the story are my wife, my children and the ducks, and even they have assumed names.

A.J.

1

'I want it,' she said, 'I want it.'

In our brief married life, I had never known her want anything so much. We both knew that we were at a crossroads: if we did not buy this house, and all it represented, whatever we did in the future would have the stigma of second best. There would always be the thought of what might have been, and the 'if only' would follow us wherever we went.

We stood at the lakeside holding hands and dreaming dreams.

'We can't possibly afford it,' she said. A bald statement, not a question, a statement simultaneously contradicted by the way that she looked at the children rushing about, investigating everything with unconcealed delight.

'No,' I agreed, 'we can't possibly afford it. You remember we couldn't afford to get married, either.'

She smiled at me, that special heart-stopping smile, as we recalled that time, a few short years ago, when I had still been a medical student. Life then had been one long series of laughs, except that she lived and worked two hundred miles from the medical school, and it was becoming tedious hitch-hiking up and down the Great North Road every other weekend.

Each time I went to see her I would take some medical textbooks with me, but I never managed so much as to open them, even though final exams were looming ever nearer.

One Sunday morning her mother announced that she had had enough; she fixed the wedding day, and I promised my future father-in-law that not only would I take care of his daughter, I would also pass my finals.

We were doing 'eyes' at the time, and I made an appointment with the Dean to ask for permission to take two weeks off, for the honeymoon. He belonged to that generation of senior physicians who had dedicated their lives, with monastic devotion, to the hospital, and who firmly believed that all acolytes to the profession should take the same vows of poverty, chastity and obedience. To him, a career in general practice was an admission of failure.

Seated behind his desk, he peered at me over his half-moon glasses.

'Why,' he asked, 'do you need to take time off now, at this critical stage in your education?'

'To get married,' I replied in all innocence, not realising the implication of his words.

'Married, boy, married?' he repeated in disgust. 'Do you have to?'

'Oh, no, sir,' I said, somewhat taken aback by the vehemence of his reaction.

'Cancel it, then,' he barked. 'You do not have my permission to take time off so near to your final exams.' And that, so far as he was concerned, was his last word.

I walked out of his office in a turmoil, wondering which was the lesser of two evils—his wrath, or that of my prospective mother-in-law. On balance, mother-in-law could be formidable, and I had already paid for the hotel, so I just slipped away and hoped that my friends would cover my absence. I never did learn anything about eyes, and they still terrify me, no matter how many I peer hopefully into, or how many books I read about them.

The dean had never noticed my absence, the honeymoon had been marvellous, and on our return I had bashed the books with an intensity that I had not believed possible. Our combined income was twenty-four pounds per calendar month, and the rent of our flat was twenty-six pounds per four-week month. We lived happily on the wrong side of Micawber's sixpence, quite sure that something would turn up, and somehow it always did.

Living beyond our income would be nothing new.

'Do you think,' my wife started to say, 'that if we economised . . .' but I finished it off for her. 'Yes, let's go and haggle over the price.'

*   *   *

2

For the two weeks of final examinations I had had to leave London and go back to my parent university. It was all a considerable ordeal. After each session with the examiners my spirits reached new depths of depression. Once I had taken the finals my grant would stop; if I failed we should have no money at all and would not even be able to keep on our small flat. To make matters worse, the Dean was one of the external examiners at the university, and the session with him in the chair of the examining board was one of the worst half-hours of my life. He asked me, not about the common disorders that I had swotted up so assiduously, but about the rare and exotic variations of his own speciality that were only mentioned in the small print of the larger textbooks.

He had treated my friend Sam just the same, and we were a miserable pair that night. Sam had deferred getting married until after he qualified; the wedding was all arranged, poised at the starting gate, to proceed if he passed and be cancelled if he failed. After his humiliating ordeal with the Dean, he phoned his fiancée and told her to cancel.

Certain in the knowledge that we had both failed, we went through the remainder of the exams more or less mechanically. Confirmation of our defeat would be a formality. The results were due to be posted on the Senate House notice board at six-thirty a.m.

I was still fast asleep in bed when Sam burst into my room at six thirty-five. 'Wake up! We're bloody doctors!' he shouted at me. 'Have a drink.' Producing a half-bottle of whisky from his back pocket, he poured two generous dollops into the tooth mugs on the wash basin. I woke up, fast.

'Are you sure?' I asked, disbelievingly. 'Have you been to look?'

'Of course,' he replied, taking a large swig of what was obviously not his first drink of the day. 'Drink that up, and come and see for yourself.'

I drank it as I dressed, neat out of the tooth mug, and we ran to the Senate House. It was true.

3

'The following candidates have satisfied the examiners,' the notice read, and there followed a list of names: ours were both there. It was far too early for breakfast, so we went back to the tooth mugs and finished off the bottle.

The rest of the morning is hazy, but I remember sitting on the floor of a public call box, completely unable to stand, with my legs stretched up against the door. I recall just being able to reach the telephone dial with the tip of one finger, and with enormous difficulty dialling O for the operator, and then asking for a reverse-charge call to Ruth.

I heard her answer and the operator say, 'Doctor Jackson is calling from a Cambridge call box. Will you pay for the call?' Then she started to cry. Eventually she said 'yes', but she had received the message. I was too drunk to speak, and she was too full of emotion.

I have no recollection of the train journey back, but I remember the evening. That was the night she became pregnant.

*   *   *

And now we had four, rushing about the garden, already declaring it home. 'I want it,' she said again, 'I want it.' And so did I, more than anything in the world.

We walked up the garden from the lake towards the house. It was an old manor house, extensively rebuilt in Georgian times, and standing in six acres of ground. Part of the garden was a moat-shaped lake, with a bridge to the island in the centre. To live here represented a way of life forever denied us in our present establishment.

Living in the town, with the surgery and waiting room taking up the front of the house, had initially seemed stimulating, but as the practice grew, it made more and more demands on us, to the extent that we were now barely able to cope with it. The telephone rang incessantly, and the population was becoming more demanding.

'It's your own fault,' Mac said to me one day, when I was grumbling to him about it. 'If you live above the shop, you're expected to be open all hours.' He was the senior partner, the original dour Scot, who had spent a life-time training his patients exactly as he wanted them. He had not got an army of retired gentlefolk ringing every evening with an up-to-date bulletin on their bowel movements, but somehow I had acquired one.

'You'll have to be firmer with them,' he told me. 'The better the service that you provide, the more it will be used. And the more it is used, the more it will be abused.'

He was quite right. I was too soft with them.

'You find yourself a nice house somewhere, and we'll build a brand new surgery.'

It was easier said than done. For months we had been looking, but had never seen anything that we fancied, or could afford. I had even asked old Jimmy Sproat to find one for me.

Jimmy was one of the regular bedtime callers, who fondly imagined that I was constantly agog to know the state of his constipation and must be informed of every development. Although not born a gentleman, he was a very astute trader, and had made enough quick money to retire early and consider himself one. Retirement had been boring, so he had set up as an estate agent, and made even more money.

He suffered from piles, and from a very real phobia that they were the harbinger of bowel cancer. Every time his piles bled, he would come to the surgery for confirmation that no cancer had developed.

I had examined him many, many times, and every year or so he had another barium enema X-ray, and a sigmoidoscopy examination. Whenever we met him at some social function, he always made a point of informing me of the state of play.

Some months before, at such a gathering, he had come up to me, drink in hand, and announced that 'they' were bleeding again. I happened to be in conversation with several other people at the time.

Thinking that I would cure him of this delightful habit, I had said to him, 'Drop your trousers and let's have a look, then,' and it was not until he had undone his belt, and his trousers were half-way down, that he had realised where he was. It had not made the slightest difference; he never

5

took the hint.

He had come to the surgery again that morning with his usual complaint, and once more I passed the proctoscope up his fundamental orifice to view his piles. He lay trouser-less on his side on the couch, while I, half-kneeling on the floor, peered up the cheeks of his behind.

'I've found your house, Doc,' he said.

'What house?' I asked, having completely forgotten that I had requested him to look out for one for me. I was far more interested in the disquieting appearance of a small ulcer just above his piles.

I withdrew the proctoscope and put my finger in. I could definitely feel the ulcer, a hard ring on the soft anal wall. It was the cancer he had been dreading for so long. He would have to have an urgent appointment with the surgeon. If I told him what it was, he would demand the operation that afternoon; it was Saturday and my afternoon off, and the surgeon certainly would not see him until Monday, not even privately.

'You've got a bit of a raw patch up there,' I told him. 'Just to make sure it's nothing, I'll get the surgeon to look at it next week.'

'OK,' he said, utterly unperturbed. 'I've arranged for you to see the house at two o'clock. You want to get in there quick. The chap who's selling is a friend of mine, and he only put it on the market this morning. The tax man's after him, and he's got to get out of the country fast. I've told him the price you'll give him, and don't you offer him a penny more. He'll settle this afternoon for a quick sale.'

'But I haven't got that sort of money,' I said, 'and never will have.'

'Look, Doc,' he replied, 'let me give you a piece of advice. Free. Inflation is just taking off. A doctor's salary will always keep up with inflation. If you buy this house now, and mortgage half your income to pay for it, in five years' time that mortgage will only be a quarter of your income, and in ten years' time will be less than ten per cent. Besides, that figure is cheap and, mark my words, house prices are going to rocket in the next few months.'

'OK,' I said, 'I'll go and see it this afternoon, just to

please you, and I'll let you know as soon as I've fixed up for you to see the surgeon again.'

He went off quite cheerfully, little knowing what was in store for him, and I continued with my surgery, little dreaming just what was in store for me.

I finished off, went to do the few visits that had come in, transferred all telephone calls to Mac and declared it my weekend off. As we sat down to lunch, I told Ruth all about Jimmy Sproat's cancer and his theory of house purchase. 'He must be right,' I said, 'because I suppose that's how he's become rich. Oh, by the way, he's made us an appointment to go and see it at two o'clock.'

'You are dreadful,' she replied. 'I reminded you at breakfast that it's Andrew's birthday. We can't possibly go anywhere this afternoon, let alone look at houses we don't want and can't afford. There's about thirty children coming at four, and I've still got all the cakes and jellies to make.'

My memory. The party had been arranged for weeks, and all conversation in the house throughout that time had been nothing but the party, and which child could ask which of his friends; yet it had gone completely from my mind when I had agreed to see the house.

As usual, I was in a mess. 'Please,' I begged. 'If we rush lunch and pile all the kids in the car, we can be there by two. We can have a quick gallop round it, say we don't want it, and then I'll help you get ready for the party.'

Against her better judgement she had agreed to come, taken one look at the house, the lake and the garden, and fallen hopelessly in love with the whole concept.

'I want it,' she said again, as we walked into the house. All the time we were sitting talking to the owners, the children ran about, exploring and deciding who should have which bedroom. At about half-past three, the owner said that he had another appointment. We stared at each other, horrified. We had all forgotten the birthday party.

We raced home and set about clearing up the lunch table. The party was a roaring success. Never had so many kids had such fun throwing flour and currants at each other as they made the party cakes, and then eating the resultant mess, dipped with their fingers in a saucepan of hot custard.

Sitting among the wreckage, there was only one topic of conversation. We had agreed to buy the house before we left, and now the problems would start. Dreams, dreams, dreams. We brushed away the problems; it was all possible.

2

I looked at the children, all on their best behaviour, sitting in a row on the chairs lining the wall. We were in the solicitor's office, all ready to sign on the dotted line, to commit ourselves to the house of our dreams and the biggest mortgage in the world.

I was terrified, it seemed such a gigantic step to take, although no one else seemed worried. But then it was St George's Day, our wedding anniversary and little George's birthday. As good a day for signing as any.

After his operation, Jimmy Sproat had rushed round organising surveyors, building societies and insurance companies. Mac had agreed quite casually and naturally that we should begin looking for somewhere to build a new surgery, and Ruth and the children were in seventh heaven.

It seemed as if I was the only one who had doubts about our ability to pay.

'Do you remember that night we first met?' asked the solicitor. 'I remember it only too well,' I replied. It had been quite an experience.

'Yes,' recalled the solicitor, 'that was rather a dirty trick to play on you.'

He, too, looked across at my family, and sighed. 'You know, one measures the passing years by the growth of children.'

The boys smiled shyly back at him and wriggled selfconsciously in their seats. George, the youngest boy and four years old today, squirmed with embarrassment as the solicitor gazed at him. 'He was less than a day old, wasn't he?'

I was surprised that the solicitor should recall the incident so clearly. It must have been on his mind all these years.

'Yes,' he repeated, 'it was a dirty trick to play on you.'

My mind wandered back to that night. It was one of our

9

wedding anniversaries I should not forget.

Ruth had gone into labour very early in the morning, and George had been born about breakfast time. The weather was foul, and the whole town seemed to be suffering from coughs and colds. Half of them had turned up for the morning surgery, and it seemed that the other half had waited until evening, when I was at my lowest ebb.

A good lady, Mrs Bunn, had been recruited to do for us, and to answer the telephone while I was out, but she had gone home hours ago.

Somehow, I got through that mammoth surgery and, opening the waiting room door, called in the last patient.

It was the solicitor, who had waited for me to see all the patients before he dropped his bombshell. He introduced himself and, as I asked him to sit down and tell me all about it, said, 'This isn't a medical matter,' and handed me a subpoena and a five-pound note.

'This says that you have to be in Stafford County Court at eleven o'clock tomorrow morning. The money is for the fare.'

I stared at him aghast.

'But I can't,' I said. 'My wife is upstairs in bed, with a baby born this morning. I can't just walk out and leave her, with two other small children as well. Besides, we've only been here for eleven weeks, and I can't abandon the practice just like that.'

'I'm afraid you'll have to,' he replied. 'That is a subpoena that has been legally handed to you.'

'Well, I'm sorry,' I said, 'I just can't go. You'll have to tell them that I am not coming, and that's all there is to it.'

'It's not as simple as that,' he told me. 'You have been formally subpoenaed to appear as a witness at Stafford County Court at eleven o'clock tomorrow morning, and failure to attend will incur a penalty of fourteen days' gaol for contempt of court.'

'Do you really mean that?' I asked. 'Look, if I've got to be in Stafford by eleven in the morning, I've got to leave tonight. However am I going to find someone to look after my wife and family and make arrangements for the morning surgery?'

10

'I'm afraid that's your problem,' he said, 'but if you're not there, you will get fourteen days.' He produced a piece of paper from his pocket. 'Would you please sign this receipt for the money and I'll leave you in peace to make your arrangements.'

Dumbstruck, I signed and he walked out.

I took the money and document upstairs to Ruth and told her all about it. She read it, and then said, 'It's no good, you'll have to go. I'm sure, if you asked her, Mrs Bunn would come back and spend the night with me, and Mac will have to look after the surgery.'

There seemed no alternative, so I 'phoned Mac and explained. 'It all happened nearly two years ago,' I told him. 'I was the houseman on the ward, when this chap was admitted with very severe jaundice. He was only a young man, and his own doctor suspected that he might have Weil's disease because apparently the ratcatchers had been round the factory where he worked, and had laid all the dead rats on his bench.'

'Sounds logical,' said Mac, 'that's the way it's usually caught.'

'Anyway,' I continued, 'his jaundice got rapidly worse, his kidneys failed, and he died. The only trouble is, I was the only one there at the time. The consultant was away, the registrar was off sick, and I had to cope by myself. I gave him everything in the book, but it was hopeless; he was dead in three days. All the tests were negative, but in spite of that, I was sure it was Weil's disease and that's what I put on his death certificate.'

'That seems straightforward enough,' Mac said. 'What's the court case all about?'

'His widow and his union are suing his employers for negligence,' I told him. 'They say it was negligent to put dead rats on his bench, and the factory say that he didn't die of Weil's disease at all, he just had a nasty case of jaundice.'

'So you're the key witness,' said Mac. 'What do the pathology boys say about it?'

'I don't honestly know,' I replied. 'You see, I came to the end of my term of office soon afterwards, and went on to the obstetric job. I never thought a word about it, until about a year ago when the union's solicitor asked me if I would give evidence for them. I was between jobs then, and it was being heard in the local town, so I said that I would. They wrote to me later, saying that the case had been postponed, and about three months ago I had another letter saying it had been postponed again. I wrote back, saying that as I had now moved and circumstances had changed, I was no longer interested. I had completely forgotten about it, till this solicitor walks into the surgery with his subpoena.'

'You'll have to go,' Mac said. 'I'll look after the patients, and you get back as soon as you can.'

Mrs Bunn was a brick. She agreed to come and look after the family, at less than five minutes' notice. I 'phoned the station and discovered that the only way to be in Stafford by eleven was to catch the next train to London, where it arrived at one a.m., and then take the six o'clock out of Euston, arriving at eight-thirty. No other trains would get me there in time.

Frantically, I threw some clothes into a suitcase, kissed my wife and Mrs Bunn goodbye and set off for the station. Mercifully, there was a solitary London taxi hanging disconsolately round Liverpool Street Station when I got there, and I asked him to take me to a hotel as near to Euston as possible, one that would give me a bed to lie on between the hours of two and six a.m. He did, and I was very grateful, and they called me in time to catch my train.

The journey up to Stafford was very dreary, nor was there much happening on Stafford Station at that hour of the morning. Wandering miserably up the platform, wondering how I was going to pass the time, I saw a man I knew get off the train. We seized on each other like long-lost friends. He was the consultant pathologist from the old hospital, up in Stafford on the same business as myself.

'What are you going to do till eleven?' I asked him, hoping that he would have something positive in mind. He had.

'Go and get some coffee at the hospital,' he replied. 'An

old friend of mine is pathologist there, and I've arranged to spend the time with him. Would you like to come as well?'

'Yes, please,' I said, and we took a taxi. On the way we discussed the case. He produced the hospital notes. None of his tests had shown the slightest sign of the spirochaetes that cause Weil's disease, nor had he been able to demonstrate any antibody to the disease in the patient's blood. The only thing that favoured a *post mortem* confirmation of Weil's disease was the microscopic picture of the kidneys. The massive damage shown there was unlikely to have been produced by the hepatitis virus, although it was not impossible.

'What do you really think?' I asked him. 'Have I made a fool of myself putting Weil's on the certificate, causing all this litigation unnecessarily?'

He thought for a moment before he replied. 'No, but Weil's is going to be impossible to prove. *I* think it was Weil's, and shall say so in court, but you know the factory have engaged the Home Office Pathologist, and by the time he's finished with us, you and I are going to look very stupid if we try to prove that's what it was.'

His friend was an absolutely splendid little man, almost perfectly spherical. He spoke with a very heavy Middle-European accent, and I did not catch his name. It had at least five syllables, and ended in something like '-inski'.

He produced some superb coffee and some spicy little cakes. I told him the story of my last-minute rush and he looked at me in horror.

'You are going into court vizout any preparation. Zat is bad, very bad. You come viz me.' He took me into his office, sat me at his desk and produced three large medical tomes. Placing the patient's hospital notes on top of the books, he commanded, 'You vill read your own notes till you haf zem by heart. Zen you vill open ze books and read everysing zere is about Veil's disease. My friend and I haf sings to do. My secretary vill bring you coffee.' And there they left me, to learn all about Weil's disease and wonder how my wife was getting on.

Just before eleven I was rescued and escorted to the court. After hanging around for an hour or so, we were

13

informed that the previous case had over-run, and our case would not be called until at least four o'clock, more likely not until the next morning.

Back to the hospital we went, and after a pint of beer and a superb pub lunch, I was once more seated at the desk, to do my preparation all over again.

Come four o'clock, the court was still not ready. The solicitor for the union introduced himself and took me off to be interviewed by the barrister acting for them. They took me through the whole sequence of events, from the initial 'phone call from the general practitioner, through every word that I had written in the notes, right up to the patient's death.

On leaving them, I met the patient's widow in the corridor. I had remembered her as a tearful young wife with three small children. It had been very painful trying to help her through her husband's deterioration, and she had been devastated by his death. She was now a prematurely old woman, not the pretty girl I remembered. Her looks had gone; she was very thin, and she wore the same coat she had worn when visiting her husband. It looked very shabby and threadbare. Very tentatively she came up to me and said, 'I never thanked you for all you tried to do for my husband. I'm sorry all this has come up. I didn't want the union to do it, but they insisted. It all seems so unnecessary and unpleasant.' And with a pathetically sad dignity she walked off alone down the corridor.

As I watched her retreating figure, I was aware that the union solicitor had come up beside me. 'She didn't want us to continue,' he said. 'The barrister doesn't think we've got a cat in hell's chance, but it's a point of principle. The members pay their dues just for eventualities like this. By the way, send your account in to the union,' and he gave me a card with the name and address on it.

For the first time, I realised that I should be paid a professional fee for my appearance in court. 'Don't forget your expenses,' he added.

'For the disturbance you've caused me,' I told him, thinking of my own wife and family, and wondering how they would cope if left in the same circumstances as the

14

widow, 'I'm going to send you a very large bill, and if I've got to hang around here all tomorrow as well, those expenses are going to be astronomical.'

Eventually we were all summoned into court and sat around, waiting for the judge. The court usher ordered us to our feet as the judge entered, and commanded us to resume our seats after the appropriate ceremonial.

I had never been involved in court proceedings before and watched it all in fascination. The outcome was immaterial to me. I had stated that in my opinion the patient had died of Weil's disease, but I held no deep conviction and was quite prepared to be over-ruled by wiser councils, if they felt that hepatitis was the correct diagnosis.

The poor chap was dead; nothing would bring him back. I felt that it was totally academic whether the cause of his massive liver and kidney failure was the Weil's spirochaete or the hepatitis virus; my sympathies were with the widow.

The barrister for the union rose and explained to the judge that we were all assembled to prove that the deceased had died of Weil's disease, as the direct result of the negligence of the factory owners who should therefore pay substantial damages to the widow.

He proposed, on this evening of the first day, to call the widow as the first witness; he would then proceed to the medical evidence, as he had no wish to detain the doctors for another whole day. A sentiment I wholly approved of; I had no desire to stay for another whole day, either.

The widow was called and very hesitantly climbed the steps into the witness box. She looked so small, so defenceless and so terribly old and haggard, that it seemed an act of criminal malice to subject her to this public ordeal.

Very gently, and with considerable courtesy and sympathy, the barrister established the basics of names, dates and places. The distress that it caused her to relive her husband's illness was evident to the whole court.

She described how he had appeared to have the 'flu, and how, instead of improving, he had relentlessly deteriorated until he had suddenly turned a bright yellow colour, become delirious and needed urgent admission to

15

hospital.

The barrister thanked her gravely and sat down. As he did so, the counsel for the factory stood up to question her. I had not noticed him before, but took an instant dislike to him. He was tall, with very straight fair hair; he was unhealthily fat—the sort of flabby fat caused by over-eating and lack of exercise—which gave his skin that greasy, shiny look that, combined with rimless spectacles and a supercilious expression, reminded me of photo-graphs of Himmler.

She was helpless and pleading for mercy. He gave her neither help nor mercy. With cold, clinical skill, he cruci-fied her, slowly, deliberately and with malice.

I watched, horrified. I did not believe that one human being could do this to another, so publicly and with such evident satisfaction. To him, she was just a pawn in the power game between big business and the union. Her feel-ings and the wreckage of her life were irrelevant. It was not the fact that he had to discredit her that dismayed and angered me, it was the evident pleasure he got from doing it.

His technique was direct and simple. An innocuous-sounding question that demanded the simple answer 'yes', followed by another, not so innocuous, and 'You have already admitted that . . .'

He left no stone unturned that could possibly be used in the defence. In case it was proved to be Weil's disease, a disease transmitted by rats, he turned her admission that she lived on a new, clean housing estate and had a small garden shed, into a confession that she lived in the equiv-alent of a gipsy encampment, on the edge of a rubbish tip, the whole over-run and infested by rats.

He made personally vicious his attack on the morals and habits of her late husband and, although I knew it to be patently untrue, I heard her admit that he was dirty, alco-holic and of sexually dubious persuasion, all of which pre-disposed to jaundice.

By the time he had finished with her she was admitting anything, anything, so that she could escape from that public humiliation. Anything to stop that ruthless

16

inquisition.

He made her admit that greed was her only motive in bringing the case, and that her husband would probably have lived, had she not been so neglectful and uncaring; that it was she herself who should have been in the dock, accused of negligence.

I had never seen anyone so mercilessly and unnecessarily destroyed. She would relive that scene, waking and sleeping, for an eternity, crying in her dreams for help that never came. Her nightmares would begin as she left that witness box and stumbled from the room.

A chill silence descended over the court.

The court usher cleared his throat and called my name. I climbed the steps into the witness box. No matter if she won the case, no matter how much money she was awarded, it could never compensate for that humiliation and degradation.

I looked down on that lawyer and hated him with a deep, unreasoning and cold hatred, of him and everything that he stood for. I watched the Home Office Pathologist move over and sit behind him. I had an intense desire to humiliate him, as he had humiliated that poor, defenceless woman. I have never, before or since, been so coldly angry.

It suddenly became imperative that I prove to the court that her husband had died of Weil's disease. If I had been at an unemotional medical meeting, discussing the case, I should probably have agreed that the weight of evidence favoured a diagnosis of hepatitis, but this was not an unemotional medical meeting, it was a court of law.

If it was justice for that barrister to do what he had just done, then it was justice to prove that those who paid him to do it had been criminally negligent in causing the death of her husband.

I had never realised before that the witness box is raised up in the air and right next to the judge's chair, so that it is quite possible to have a personal and private conversation with him and be oblivious of the rest of the court. The barristers' bench was some distance away, so that they had to shout up at me and I could look down on them, giving my answers directly to the judge in a conversational voice. A position of great inherent superiority.

I looked down on the greasy blond man and he looked up at me, and neither of us liked what we saw.

The first questions from the union's barrister were factual and straightforward: dates, times, clinical findings and so on. It struck me quite forcibly as he went through the chronological sequence, that I was the only doctor in the hospital who had examined the patient while he was still alive. My written notes were gospel, there was no one who could refute them.

I told the judge that clinically there could be no doubt that the patient had died of Weil's disease. I told him of the first telephone call from the general practitioner who had been the first to make the diagnosis on the basis of the rats at work, and on the clinical progress of the disease. I also added that I had a great respect for that man who, although he was not in court, was a very experienced ex-army doctor whose opinions were not lightly to be ignored. Although not actually stating it, I conveyed the deliberate impression that he had considerable experience of Weil's disease.

As an aside, I tossed in the fact that I, too, had been a GP working in the same area, which I knew well. The housing estate in which the patient had lived was a new, clean council estate, without a rat in sight.

I also told him how the widow had sat beside her husband's bed for the whole three days, devotedly caring for him.

The judge nodded his agreement as if he, too, had been distressed by the treatment of the widow.

Greasy Yellowhair stood up and went straight into the attack. He used exactly the same tactics as he had used on the widow. He intended to demolish me in exactly the same way, in as short a time as possible.

The Home Office Pathologist whispered instructions into his back. He began to ask me questions about the white cell count in the patient's blood.

Thanks to my morning spent with the books, and having watched his methodical and brutal treatment of the

18

widow, I realised exactly where his questions were leading.

The disturbance in the composition of the various types of white blood cells had been non-specific, a slight decrease in all the constituent forms. This is quite typical of hepatitis. Weil's disease should have shown an increase in the leucocytes. He wanted me to admit this or, better still, that I was ignorant on this point—as, in fact, I had been until that morning—and I thanked my guardian angel for little 'Five-syllables-inski' and his insistence on doing my preparation. One of his books had stated quite clearly that in fatal cases of Weil's disease the whole blood picture is one of depression of all forms, and only in those cases likely to recover is the leucocyte count raised.

I answered the questions, quoting from memory great chunks of the book as I did so, explaining why the figures, which at first sight seemed to indicate quite clearly that the man had suffered from hepatitis, were in fact quite compatible with a diagnosis of Weil's disease. As I expounded, with the fire of emotion and the confidence of newly acquired knowledge, I found that I was talking directly to the judge and explaining it to him alone.

Prompted by the Home Office, Greasy Yellowhair kept interrupting our conversation with more questions, the angling of which was obvious. Arrogantly, I brushed them aside. Each one I answered needed only a simple 'yes', but I then went on to explain why the answer could be 'no', and in so doing gave him the answer to the next question he was about to ask, and why this was also 'no'.

It threw him completely off balance, so that he lost his thread, and his confidence. I was enjoying myself enormously, and the judge appeared to be enjoying it, too. He smiled at me and nodded his head frequently, encouraging me to go on as I made that barrister look more and more incompetent and inept.

Greasy Yellowhair abandoned blood and started asking about the causative spirochaete of Weil's disease. 'Did you find any in the patient's blood?' he asked. The straight answer was 'no', from which it would follow that the patient could not have had the disease.

19

'But,' I explained to the judge, 'there were none in the sample of blood sent to the path lab because I'd killed them. The patient was admitted late at night, with what seemed to me to be an obvious case of Weil's disease. He was severely ill, and the whole object of my actions that night was to save his life, not to prove my diagnosis in a court of law two years later. The GP had started treatment and I set up a drip and gave him the maximum possible dose of the recommended antibiotic, directly into a vein, every four hours. This was effective in killing all the spiro-chaetes, but the damage that they had already done to his liver and kidneys was too great for him to recover.'

The judge nodded encouragingly.

'The sample of blood sent to the lab next morning could not possibly have contained any spirochaetes,' I said. In fact I had no idea how long the spirochaetes, if any, would have persisted after the first dose of antibiotic.

Greasy Yellowhair spluttered in indignation and the Home Office Pathologist jumped up and down in grave displeasure, but the judge agreed with every word I said.

Next came the question of antibodies. 'Were there any in his blood?' counsel asked. Again, the straight answer was 'no', and again it could not possibly be proved to be Weil's disease in their absence. But what applied to the missing leucocytes could also apply to the missing antibodies.

I explained to the judge exactly why, in my opinion, there were no antibodies. 'You see, Your Honour,' I said, 'antibodies are the body's defence against infection. Where the body puts up a good fight, it makes defences, and as the illness progresses and the person recovers, these antibodies can be detected and measured. The nearer to complete recovery, the greater the amount found in the blood. But in this case, the infection was overwhelm-ing, and the poor chap did not have time to make any anti-bodies. There were no antibodies in his blood because he didn't have any. He was overwhelmed and killed by an infection to which he had no resistance.'

The judge smiled at me and nodded sagely. Although made up on the spur of the moment, it certainly sounded good, but it was too much for the Home Office Pathologist.

Prodding Greasy Yellowhair vigorously in the back, he said in a very loud whisper, audible throughout the court, 'Ask him on what evidence he bases that statement,' and Greasy Yellowhair obliged.

I looked blankly at the judge and he looked encouragingly back. I did not have any evidence: there was none. 'It's common medical knowledge,' I stated eventually, which, thinking about it afterwards, was unanswerable.

'Ask him where he qualified,' came the stage whisper.

'I hold a Cambridge medical degree,' I told the judge, 'but I did my clinical training at one of the London teaching hospitals.' This, too, was unanswerable, and I stood down feeling completely victorious. I had avenged my patient's widow.

The pathologist followed me into the box and was detained there for only a few minutes. He explained all his equivocal results, but thought that the microscope slides of the kidneys were diagnostic of Weil's disease. Greasy Yellowhair had no questions and the court adjourned for the day.

The union solicitor came up to me and shook my hand warmly. 'That was magnificent,' he said. 'You have won the case for us. You should have raised the ante.'

For a moment, I did not understand what he was saying, then I realised that he was telling me to raise my fee. 'I just did,' I replied, 'and your expenses are going to include a first-class hotel for tonight.'

'Make 'em as big as you like,' he replied. 'After your performance tonight, the other side will be paying. No questions asked.'

'Do you really mean that?' I asked suspiciously.

'Wouldn't have said it if I didn't,' he replied. 'We were thinking of withdrawing after the widow had got so badly minced, and if you'd been minced up as well, I'd have been in that judge's office now, trying to avoid paying the other side's expenses.'

'I wouldn't have done it,' I told him, 'if he hadn't taken such obvious delight in torturing that poor woman. I saw the other side, you know. I had to hold her hand for three days, while he lay dying.'

21

'I know,' he said, 'the union's done the same since.'

'Where is she?' I asked. 'I would just like to say goodbye.'

'She's gone,' he said, nodding at the open door. 'My secretary took her straight home in my car. I've got to catch the train.'

'Please give her my regards,' I said as he walked away.

The court room had emptied magically while we had been talking. There was no one else there to say goodbye to, so I took a lonely taxi to the station and, at some ungodly hour the next morning, arrived home and crept into bed without waking my wife or the baby.

After surgery, I made up a bill for a fee of one hundred guineas, and nearly as much for expenses, duly and fraudulently itemised.

It was paid a few days later. The letter accompanying the cheque pointed out that the recognised fee for someone of my lowly medical status was seven pounds, with four more a day for expenses. It also stated that I had charged more than the Home Office Pathologist, but in view of the outcome, they were happy to enclose the opposition's cheque.

The widow had been awarded a very substantial sum.

*   *   *

Now, four years later, I sat in the office of the solicitor who had started it all, day-dreaming, savouring the memory. Day-dreaming of St George slaying dragons, and of damsels rescued from distress.

Little George wanted to go to the toilet. The solicitor was saying something.

'Sign here, and here, both of you.'

We signed.

'You may take possession on May the twenty-ninth.'

We walked out of that office on air. There were only four weeks to wait.

3

'The gift of sight is a wondrous thing,' Herbert Allcock would declaim, 'and let us praise the Lord for it.'

He praised the Lord for many other things besides sight, and it was characteristic of the man that, by normal standards, he had very poor vision and a terrible squint.

Born just before the turn of the century, somewhere in the middle of a very large family not overblessed with either industry or intelligence, Herbert had somehow grown up and got along, but he was so short-sighted that he was chronically accident-prone.

If anyone fell in the harbour, it was Herbert. If someone went too near a horse and got kicked, it was Herbert. By adolescence he had, at one time or another, broken most of the bones in his body. The whole family, including himself, treated his clumsiness as a huge joke. They swept him through life in their midst, partially protecting him from it; there was always someone to pick up the pieces.

By the time that he obtained a pair of glasses his eyesight had become very poor. He suffered from a condition called progressive myopia in which the initial short sight gets progressively worse, so that anything further than a few inches from his nose was so out of focus as to be just a vague blur. Movement was all he could detect.

His left eye was much more afflicted than his right, so that it was patently true when he said, 'I use my right eye for distance and my left for close-up.'

What he failed to say was that, to see at all, he needed enormous pebble lenses in front of each eye, and the eye he was not using turned towards his nose to such an extent that only the white was visible. Since the power of binocular vision had been lost in early infancy, any attempt at correcting his squint, although it would have made him cosmetically more acceptable, would have given him very troublesome double vision and, probably, severe headaches, too, until he redeveloped his squint.

It was this lack of sight that almost certainly saved his life during the Great War. When Lord Kitchener called for his second volunteer army, all his brothers and friends enlisted as a gang, with Herbert smuggled somewhere in the middle. Ages were falsified, where necessary, and Herbert's disability disguised. He was discharged after a few weeks, when they discovered that he was virtually blind.

Not one of the others survived the Somme.

Herbert spent the war apprenticed to an old cobbler. 'It was that or tailoring,' he told me once, 'and I just couldn't see myself sitting cross-eyed and cross-legged on a bit of cloth all day, cutting out waistcoats.'

With his leather a few inches from his nose, under the guidance of the old cobbler he learned eventually how to make a very creditable pair of boots.

Boot-mending became his living, but fish-breeding was his joy. He lived in an old Victorian terraced house, two rooms on each floor, but three stories high. The ground floor was his workshop, and the family lived above. His was the end house of the terrace, and his large garden merged into the builder's yard next door. It was difficult to define the boundary, as his garden was not a garden in the accepted sense, but a collection of fishponds. Some were concreted holes in the ground, some were cut-down oil tanks partially buried, and many defied description. Any container that held water also held fish, or had water plants growing in it.

In places, Herbert had overflowed into the builder's yard and, in others, the builder's yard had flowed back. Tanks and ponds cohabited peacefully with piles of bricks, heaps of old timber, mountains of rubble and the assorted junk of ages belonging to both parties.

It was a positive death-trap to the unwary but, from tending his fish twice daily, Herbert knew every inch of the way.

The house inside was equally chaotic. The walls of the front showroom were lined with fish-tanks of many shapes and sizes, all festooned with heating wires and air

24

lines. Some held tropical fish, and some held cold-water species. Since Herbert did all his tropical fish-breeding in the front room, he kept his fish food there, too: water fleas from a smelly duck pond, thin redworms specially garnered from the mud round the sewage works, and jars of infusoria, all mixed in with the fish for sale. Scattered among them were the tanks containing his breeding pairs of fish.

The infusoria were his special culture, produced by many years of devoted effort. Infusoria are microscopic aquatic creatures that live on the rotting vegetation at the bottom of ponds. They are ideal as the first food of newly-hatched fish which are themselves only just big enough to see with the naked eye. Close up, Herbert could see them clearly, and spent many hours watching them when he should have been mending shoes. The infusoria culture was essentially an old sweet jar, with a lettuce—roots, soil and all—rotting under water. Several times a day Herbert would take a teaspoonful of the culture to feed his baby fish. He would top up the level of the sweet jar each time until the aroma reached a certain pitch, when the lettuce inside was replaced with a fresh one.

The secret of fish-breeding, he told me, was knowing when to change the lettuce. 'If you change it too soon, then the brew is too thin and all your little fish will starve. If you leave it too long, other things will grow, that will kill your fish. Smell that now, boy. That's just right. Save a cupful to start the new culture, and you'll never go wrong.'

Piled on old boxes, heaped on several old tables and jostling with the fish for space, were the shoes awaiting collection. Happily mixed in with them were tins of boot polish, advertisments for leather and new and second-hand army boots.

The pairs were tied together by the laces, with the price, or the charge, written on a bit of paper stuffed into one of the toes. Herbert stoutly maintained that, as all his customers knew their own footwear, there was no necessity to write their names as well. The truth was that, although he could read, writing was an almost impossible task. At least half the bits of paper had parted company from their shoes, as customers rummaged among the piles to find their footware. It was a standing joke that everyone tried to get a better pair of shoes than the ones that they had brought in, but nobody ever did.

The back room was worse than the front. In its centre was a large bench to which was attached his last, and an enormous sewing machine worked by a treadle. The entire bench was covered with bits of leather, rubber soles and heels, the tools of his trade, and much assorted junk several inches deep. On top of that lay all the work in hand—shoes, fish tanks, broken garden gnomes, all patiently waiting their turn. The chaos never bothered him; if it was more than six inches from his nose, he could not see it.

There was just enough space in the room to walk the two steps to his stool. The rest was filled from floor to ceiling with a lifetime's accumulation. Partially opened bags of cement, aquarium angle iron, an old central heating system never installed, shoes and rubbish. Fresh possessions were piled on the top, together with new stocks of boots, until they, too, were lost.

The slowly-rising tide of junk overflowed up the stairs and into the living quarters. In the midst of it all Herbert was content. 'Praise the Lord,' he'd say, 'that I can still earn a living.' Somehow, among it all, he and his wife had conceived, borne and reared nine children. None of them had been remotely interested in either fish or shoes, and all had left home to do their own thing. Herbert had praised the Lord for their birth, and again for their departure.

His transport was an old motor bike, to which was attached a side-car and various other containers. For many years he had successfuly conveyed his family, his fish and all their impedimenta many hundreds of miles without mishap. Even with his glasses, his forward vision was severely limited, but at thirty miles per hour, stationary objects had a relative velocity that made their movement apparent to him.

The new road system was his undoing. Without telling him, they had straightened the road and put in a new 'Keep Left' bollard. He took the corner in his usual way,

26

and wrapped his motor bike and side-car neatly round the new bollard, before the cement had even set. Mercifully his only passengers were several jars of water fleas. Herbert lost his glasses, which was catastrophic, and broke his shoulder and thigh, which was a minor nuisance. 'Praise the Lord,' he said as he came round in the ambulance, 'the wife should have been holding those fleas.'

Once his bones had been set he was allowed home from the hospital, and I had to visit him frequently to check for complications.

'Praise the Lord,' he said as he put on his new glasses, 'for the gift of sight.' Being confined to bed for several weeks was an inconvenience he accepted with complete equanimity.

The Lord Herbert praised was not the one normally found in the Book of Common Prayer. As his parents had had no time for religion—until the war, when his brothers and friends were killed—he had never been in a church in his life. Their departure had left a tremendous void and, as he said, 'I had no one to pick me up when I fell.'

The old cobbler to whom he had been apprenticed was a member of an exclusive sect of brethren, and they picked him up. After work Herbert went along to the meetings, and here he found something of the fellowship that the war had taken from him. He joined in their rituals and worship with gusto. He understood little of the theology, only that there was a life after death, that alcohol and tobacco were forbidden, and that the rules of the brotherhood must be obeyed to the letter.

The form of worship that they practised was entirely to his liking, and he went night after night to the meeting house, just to enjoy it. He belted out all the hymns with great fervour, praised the Lord with all his soul and listened to the forceful prayers of the elders with the wonder and faith of the convert.

Unfortunately it did not last. The old cobbler committed some unforgivable misdemeanour, for which he was not prepared to repent in public, and was ceremonially drummed out of the brethren. His family went with him and, as Herbert counted himself as family, he had to leave,

27

too. Characteristically picking up the pieces, he and the old cobbler opened up a branch meeting house of their own at their workshop, at which they were the only worshippers. They prayed aloud and hummed the tunes together, until the old cobbler eventually died. Herbert continued to pray aloud, in public and in private, and occasionally hummed a tune. He obeyed the tenets of the brethren to the letter, particularly those on smoking and drinking.

* * *

I had been up most of the night, delivering a baby at a house not far from Herbert's. I was very tired, it had been a difficult birth and a whole day's work loomed ahead. It was about seven o'clock, and all the lights were on in his house, so I thought that I would call and see him before I went home to breakfast, and so save myself the visit later in the day.

His wife welcomed me with open arms and asked me if I would care to join them in an early starter. Assuming that she meant a cup of tea, I accepted with alacrity and went upstairs to check on Herbert. He was fine, all his plasters comfortable, no bedsores and no pain. We chatted for a few minutes about the desirability of putting fish and ornamental plants in my new lake, while we waited for his wife to bring in the tea.

It was not tea she brought in, but three large, long-stemmed glasses, full of a clear, deep-red liquid that looked just like port. I took my glass and watched Herbert and his wife knock theirs back with obvious practice and relish. Mrs Allcock looked at me enquiringly as she refilled their glasses and I took my first sip. It tasted just like port, too, with an overlying hint of something else. Very pleasant first thing in the morning, after an all-night effort. The taste eluded me, but I had the proffered second glass, and then a third. I already felt much better, and racked my brains for that elusive taste. It was fruity and autumnal, and at last it came: elderberry wine—only this was the strongest and the best that I had ever tasted.

28

'This is delicious,' I told them. 'What is it?'

'Elderberry juice,' replied Herbert. 'We have a glass of it every morning of our lives. Sometimes two or three.'

I was dying to ask him how he reconciled this potent brew with his teetotal convictions, but did not know quite how to broach the subject.

'How do you make it?' was the best I could muster.

'We do not make it,' he replied with great feeling, 'the Lord does. All we do is to gather the berries and squash them in a large jug, and then wait till the Lord has finished working on it. As soon as He's finished working, but not before, we bottle it up and then leave it for five years. The Lord takes a little time to make His best.'

'Mmm,' I said, not daring to hint that he was brewing alcohol by the oldest method known to man, 'Do you, er, use any other fruit like this?'

'Oh yes,' he replied, 'the good Lord made the fruits of the earth so that we may enjoy them. We use all sorts of fruit, vegetables, too. We never waste anything, and treat them all the same. The wife soaks them all in a great big bucket, and when they've finished working the Lord's will, we bottle them.'

I slowly digested this. 'Mother,' he said, 'take Doc through into the other room and show him our store.' I followed her into the back room. The reverence with which I was shown round indicated only too clearly that this room took the place of their own private chapel. It was impossible to move in it for bottles, stacked from floor to ceiling.

'Praise the Lord,' I said with a reverence to match Herbert's.

Every bottle was labelled. Parsnip, rhubarb, peapod, plum, and dozens of others. An enormous shelf full of bottles of urine-coloured fluid, labelled 'Orange and P', caught my eye. 'What's the P?' I asked.

'Peel,' she replied. 'Sometimes I make it with the peel still on, sometimes without. He likes it with, but that's too bitter for me, I prefer it without.' She walked up to the shelf and took down a bottle. 'Try some,' she said as she uncorked it, and poured me about half a pint. It was a tangy bitter orange, and went down well.

We went back into Herbert's room. 'You've got enough there to last a life-time,' I remarked.

'Oh no,' he said. 'Most of it has to be kept for several years, and we drink about five bottles a day. Got to keep making it in advance.'

I tried to work it out. Five bottles of that stuff a day— they were never sober. 'We have our early morning elder- berry, breakfast with the orange, and the best of all is the midmorning parsnip. Keeps you going, that does.' He thought for a minute. 'Here, if you've been up half the night, you'll need some of that,' and mother was dis- patched to fetch some.

I have had worse whisky. It burned all the way down.

Half-way through it, I suddenly felt very ill. Herbert, lying in bed, seemed to advance and recede in a most alarming manner. His voice faded away. He looked at me very anxiously, and then became two Herberts.

He reached out his good hand towards me, and as it neared me it became two hands. I blinked several times, and forced him and his hands to become one again. His voice echoed round and round. 'Are you all right, Doc?' The concern echoed after his words.

'Yes,' I said, and the rest just did not come. I was aware that my mouth was moving, but it was not connected to my vocal cords, and my whole being was floating far above this inarticulate body of mine. I stood up. At least, in theory I stood up. In fact nothing happened. I tried again. This time, my legs worked as far down as the knees and, clutching the end of Herbert's bed, I achieved the erect posture.

'I must go, or I shall be late for surgery,' I tried to say, but what came out was a meaningless slur of sound. I started for the door, but it kept moving off to the right. I stopped, executed a brilliant military right turn and set off again. The door moved even further to the right. I stopped again, did another right turn, and marched forward once more. This time the door went on moving to the right and I fol- lowed it, faster and faster, until I suddenly found myself lying face down on the floor, with Mrs Allcock peering at me from far too close. Completely out of focus, she came and went as the room revolved.

'Doctor, are you ill?'

I felt a great kinship with the babe that I had delivered that morning. He had been stuck in the position known as deep transverse arrest. I was sure I was in the same position now. There was a pair of forceps round my head, my chest was tightly constricted, and all I could do was kick my legs uselessly in a very confined space.

'Coffee,' I croaked, 'coffee.' The word came out the second time and the coffee miraculously appeared. It was hot, sweet and nearly all milk. Somehow I drank it. Great waves of something nasty rose up from my stomach into my head and back down to the stomach again. With each wave, the floor rose and fell and tipped at a most alarming angle. If I just stayed still, I thought, I would slide down the slope to the door, and then into the lavatory where I could be sick and feel much better.

Staying very still, I slid across the room, round the door and into the bathroom, where I lay on the floor, with my chin on the pedestal, and Mrs Allcock held my head to correct my aim.

Very clearly, with beautiful enunciation, a voice that sounded like mine said, 'I wish I hadn't had that coffee.'

Mac came to rescue me. I was unaware that they had sent for him, or what they had said to him, but he thought it was a huge joke. He administered some fiendish Scottish concoction and drove me home.

My surgery should have started at nine. By half-past I thought I could cope and went into the consulting room. The first patient was a small child with diarrhoea and vomiting, who gave a convincing demonstration of his troubles by puking straight into my lap, simultaneously filling his trousers with an evil smell. He caught both me and my stomach unawares, my body heaved, and I returned the compliment all over him and his mother.

Defeat was not only inevitable but immediate. I fled, leaving my poor wife to clean up the mess and somehow dispose of all the waiting patients.

That afternoon, Mrs Allcock brought round a bottle of their special stomach mixture, rhubarb tonic that they made themselves and, if the Lord be praised, I'd be better by morning.

I neither desired nor dared to open it.

4

Joshua Waterton should have been born a bull. He looked like one, and he behaved like one. He did not believe in waiting rooms or appointment systems.

I could hear him now, stomping up the hall.

His usual complaint was constipation, and I had to give him the medical equivalent of hand grenades to get him moving at all. A lifetime of fried ship's food had left his bowels permanently sluggish. All his life, as a trawler skipper, not having to take his trousers down for the two weeks he was at sea had been very convenient, but now that he had retired he had become obsessive about his lack of bowel movement. At least twice each week he would barge into the surgery, stamping all over my appointment system and, with ill-concealed impatience, would stand outside my closed surgery door.

He had such a dominant and overbearing personality that, even through a closed door, the patient of the moment was aware that Joshua Waterton was being kept waiting, and hurried up the consultation.

Once inside, it never occurred to him that he was delaying other people, and he behaved as if he had all the time in the world—which indeed he had. For him, the problems of other people paled into insignificance when confronted by the fact that he had not 'been' for three days. This was a serious emergency and, even if it had not been, the rest of the human race only existed to do his bidding, as they had done all his life. A command from him, whether to his crew or his family, was followed by instant obedience, or by being knocked senseless with one blow from his great ham fist.

* * *

Mrs Bessey, who was only suffering from a severe and

33

generalised skin rash, a neurodermatitis produced by chronic anxiety, sensed the extraordinary presence of this dominant male and, clutching her prescription for another tube of cream, scuttled from the surgery.

Bull-like, he advanced to the recently vacated chair and, banging his great knobbly stick on the desk, sat arthritically down and dominated all he surveyed. His conversation was always a monologue. He dictated the subject and what was said about it, and continued talking across anyone who had the temerity to try to interrupt.

There were only two subjects: his constipation, and the sea. Many times I had been subjected to his version of how, single-handed, he had rammed and sunk a German submarine just off Liverpool, and how the regular navy was run by a pack of spineless incompetents who could not even find the wreck, despite his specific instructions. The story of how he had guided them to it, using only the colour and direction of the waves, usually took at least forty minutes.

But today his theme was neither constipation nor the sea. Wheezing slightly, his massive chest heaving from the effort of sitting down, he put a great paw into his inside pocket and produced a piece of paper. He thumped it onto the desk, with sufficient force to make the pens in their stand rattle and my ophthalmoscope fall over and roll onto the floor. I retrieved it and anxiously checked that it was still functional. This he completely ignored. Jabbing his piece of paper with an enormous finger, he ordered, 'Read that.'

I read it. He had been summonsed to appear in court on a charge of dangerous driving.

He was a menace on the road. Having grown up in the days when sail took right of way over steam, he drove his old car as if he was still master of a clipper ship. He had the natural right of passage over everything else on the road.

The garage in which he kept his car was an old shed on the allotments adjoining the A12. He always backed straight out of this into the main road. Not believing in mirrors, and having such a rigid and arthritic spine, he could only see where he was going by lining up with his point of

34

departure until the nose of his car was clear of the gateway and he could engage forward gear. To my personal knowledge he had nearly caused several nasty accidents. I presumed someone who had just missed him had reported him to the police.

I handed him back the summons. 'Why?' I asked. 'What happened?'

'Some people just don't think.' He snorted angrily, those dominant eyes glaring at me out of that weather-beaten face, surmounted by his close-cropped, iron-grey hair. I could see just why he had been master of every vessel he had ever sailed in, and of every man he had ever met. 'For fifty years I have been coming home from the harbour and turning right into my garage. Everybody knows that I turn right there.'

Even in his old age, he certainly had a tremendous presence. Those eyes drilled into me.

'I was half-way across the road when this fool hit me full tilt up the stern, didn't he?' Angrily, he leaned forward in his chair. 'And then this other damn fool can't stop, because he's going too fast, and has to hit me up the front, didn't he?'

Mesmerised, I waited for him to continue as he breathed heavily and, quite unconsciously, held me transfixed.

'Were you hurt?' I asked eventually.

'Hurt? Of course I was damn' well hurt. That's what I've come to see you about.'

'Where?' I asked, but he ignored the interruption.

'My damned door wouldn't open, and the seat had come off. I had to stay there, hanging onto the steering wheel, like a coat on a coat hanger, didn't I? Till they cut me out.'

'Did they take you to hospital?'

'Yes, the damn' fools. They put me on this stretcher thing before I could stand up, and carted me off.'

'Did the hospital give you a letter for me?' I successfully interrupted him. The great paw went once again inside his coat, and he produced an envelope. He had not bothered to disguise the fact that he had opened it and read the letter. The envelope had been crudely ripped by one of his great fingers, and almost torn in half.

I thought of the old iron men in wooden ships. He was certainly one of them. The Casualty Officer had examined him thoroughly and X-rayed most of him. He had three fractured right ribs and his left side was severely bruised. The letter was several days old, and he had not even mentioned the pain, only anger at being done for dangerous driving.

In the fullness of time—his time—I eventually got his shirt off and inspected the damage. He was black and blue all over, those fractured ribs creaked ominously, and the bases of his lungs were quite moist.

'Does it hurt to cough?' I enquired.

'Of course it damn' well does.' The look on his face told me not to ask so many damn' fool questions.

'I'd better give you some antibiotics, to stop that setting up into a nasty chest infection,' I told him.

He regarded the prescription suspiciously. 'They won't bung me up, like the last damn' lot of pills you gave me?' he asked.

'No,' I replied, hoping that they would not. With a bit of luck, they would give him the nearest thing to diarrhoea that he had ever had.

Dressed again, and leaning heavily on his stick, he creaked his way out and I resumed my interrupted surgery.

He did not return for nearly two weeks, which was just about his record for non-attendance. As usual, he rode unknowingly roughshod over the indignant but silent opposition in the waiting room.

'Give me some more of them pills,' he commanded without preamble, and held out a massive hand for the prescription. He was obviously in a bad mood, a bull with something on its mind, proceeding through the china shop of humanity. I had something on my mind, too—the last patient—and I was trying to make a telephone call. He was not to be put off and, as I tried to dial the number, repeated, 'Give me some more of them pills. I haven't got all day.'

I waved him into the chair, while I made an urgent

appointment for the previous patient to be seen at the hospital. Surprisingly, he sat down and waited for me to finish. Barely had I replaced the telephone when he resumed, in a tone of voice that I could imagine him using to tell one of his deckhands to pass him the hammer.

'How is your chest?' I asked.

'Bloody chest's all right, but I haven't been for three days. Went every day with those pills. The best I've ever had. Why the hell didn't you give them me before?'

The antibiotic pills in question were ampicillin, one of the penicillins with a marked tendency to have the side effect of causing a nasty diarrhoea. For him to use them on a regular basis as a purgative would create more problems that it solved. The waiting room was full, and I was running very late.

'Pull up your shirt,' I ordered, in my best no-nonsense voice, and applied the end of my stethoscope to his bare chest. The broken ribs still creaked, and his bases were still very moist.

'OK,' I nodded at him. 'You can have some more. Tuck your shirt in.'

While I was writing out the prescription, he produced a letter. Angrily he thrust it at me. 'For fifty years I've had a clean record. Never had an accident, and now look at that.'

It was a letter from his insurance company, pointing out that as he had omitted to pay the previous year's premium, they had no further interest in the matter of his wrecked car, nor in the claims of the other two drivers. Not only would he be done for dangerous driving, but for being uninsured as well.

I gave him enough ampicillin for a further two weeks, to last him until after he had come up in court.

It worked. He had not returned when I saw in the local paper the banner headline, 'Local Skipper fined £250. Ordered to take Driving Test.' There followed a report of angry exchanges between him and the magistrate, and details of the indignation from both the unfortunate drivers who, unaware of where he garaged his car, had obstructed his right of way to it.

An audible silence descenced on the waiting room when

he stomped through it a few days later. Even I, behind my closed surgery door, was aware of the vibes as he waited in frustrated impatience outside it.

Waving yet another piece of paper at me as he advanced across the room, he thumped it on the desk with his usual force and ordered, 'This is where you have to sign it,' and, almost shaking with fury, waited for me to do so.

The insurance company had declined to insure him until he had a medical certificate of fitness to drive, and only then at an exorbitant premium. Not only that, but he could not take a driving test without a medical certificate, either.

'Sign it here,' in that 'pass the hammer' voice.

I could not possibly sign that he was medically fit to drive. It was the equivalent of perjury and, besides, I might be the one he hit next time.

The finger jabbed at the paper. His presence filled the room. It was very difficult not to be overpowered by that dominant personality and that bulldozing will. The feeling of being dominated was aggravated by the fact that I was still sitting in my chair while he stood, towering massively above me, the violence in him barely restrained.

Psychologically, I reversed roles. 'Sit down,' I commanded, ordering him to pass *me* the hammer, and stood up myself, towering over *him*. He sat down, an angry cornered bull, ready to charge and smash anything that looked remotely like a red rag.

'I can't sign that,' I said, as his heaving chest wheezed in anger, and he glared balefully back up at me. 'It's a legal document that says I have fully examined you, tested your reflexes and measured your eyesight. If I am going to take the responsibility of perhaps having to stand up in court and say you are fit to drive, I am going to do these things first.'

We glared at each other. He was the first to look away. Adding insult to injury, I told him, 'We have to charge a fee for the examination, whether we say you're fit to drive or not. The examination takes about half an hour. Make an appointment for it as you go out, and bring a specimen of your water with you when you come.'

Looking murderous but saying nothing, he savagely

grabbed his piece of paper and stomped out. They probably heard him two streets away as he forced the little receptionist into a verbal corner, ordering his appointment and reducing her to tearful incompetence.

He was back that afternoon. The receptionist spent most of her lunch time cancelling and rearranging her shattered appointment system. A pint beer bottle, full of his urine, landed on the desk with the force of a cannon ball. I realised now that I had made the correct decision in training to become a doctor, not a vet. Cornering and roping creatures such as this, prior to examining them, must be hard and dangerous work.

I examined him fully. His reflexes were too sluggish, his eyesight too poor and there was arthritic stiffness in his joints. All individually were sufficient reasons to fail him. Besides these, his blood pressure was nearly off the clock and his pulse very irregular, which added overtones of heart failure to his still congested lungs. There was no way that I could give him a certificate of fitness to drive. Equally, there was no way I could not, without grave risk of serious injury to myself.

I compromised, telling him that as his heart was a bit irregular, I could not give him the full fitness certificate, but would give him a letter, stating that he was fit enough to take a driving test. With this, he could arrange the appointment for his test, while the pills that I was about to give him would control the irregularity of his heart. He could have his full certificate when he had passed his driving test and his heart was back to normal.

He left the surgery, clutching a prescription for digitalis and a certificate stating that he could be safely subjected to a driving test, but making no mention of his medical fitness.

Within seconds he was back. 'Give me some more of them other pills.' I capitulated, despite the fact that he was obviously taking them a handful at a time, every third night. Enough was enough for one day. I would rejoin battle with his constipation on another occasion.

Several weeks passed, and he did not return. His absence was conspicuous. Whatever his other problems, the constipation was not bothering him.

Towards the end of one morning surgery, the reception-ist slipped in an extra patient, an emergency. 'I think he's broken his hand,' she said. He was a young man whom I had not met before, and he held out his hand for me to see. On the back of it was an enormous swollen bruise, but the bones appeared to be intact.

'How did you do that?' I asked conversationally, as I pre-pared to bind it up.

'You'll never believe it,' he replied, 'but I was hit by a gear lever.'

'What, in an accident?'

'No. You see, I'm a driving test examiner, and this old boy I was testing was so bad, that after he'd been round the wrong side of a roundabout, I told him to pull in and stop the car, and I caught hold of the steering wheel to pull him into the side. D'you know, he broke off the gear lever and hit my hand with it.'

'Not by the name of Joshua Waterton,I suppose?'

'Yes, that's him. I told him he'd failed his test, took his ignition keys, and left him on the side of the road. I walked up here. He was purple with rage, dancing up and down, when I left him. I'm going to sue him for assault and report him for dangerous driving.'

He left the surgery, suitably bandaged. I expected Joshua himself at any moment, but still he did not come. It was another good three weeks before he appeared, incred-ibly quite docile. He showed me the papers for his next court appearances, on a charge of dangerous driving again, and also of assaulting the driving examiner.

I asked him how the driving test had gone. He settled himself in the chair. 'Oh God,' I thought to myself, 'this is going to take longer than the Liverpool submarine.'

It did. The essence of his story was that as he had approached the roundabout and attempted to change gear, the gear lever had come off in his hand. Knowing that, if he stopped, he would never start again in top gear, he did the only sensible thing and dodged through the traf-fic on a short cut, displaying, in his opinion, considerable presence of mind. He had brushed aside the hand of the examiner when the latter tried to stop him, because he knew that, once stationary, he was stranded. His opinion of the examiner was not high.

I took his pulse, which was regular, listened to his chest, which was clear, and enquired about his constipation. He was taking the digitalis, not according to instructions, but again to regulate his bowels.

The therapeutic dose of digitalis is only slightly less than the toxic dose. The first symptom of digitalis overdosage is often a loose motion. Joshua was taking just enough to keep him loose, regulating his own dosage by this criterion, and quite accidentally taking the optimum dose for his heart.

I gave him another hundred. Three months of no Joshua Waterton would be unmitigated bliss.

5

I sat at my desk, waiting for the telephone to ring. Impatiently, I looked, yet again, at my watch. A full ten minutes had elapsed since I had shown Jill to the door. 'She must be home by now,' I thought.

I was beginning to worry. She was the first patient I had treated with hypnotherapy in cold blood, and I had given her the post hypnotic suggestion that she would telephone me, at the surgery, to let me know that she had arrived home safely.

There was reason for my worry. To get home, she had to cross the railway line, over the bridge. This was a perfectly ordinary road bridge, but when the road had been widened many years ago, the old pedestrian pavements had been incorporated into the newly widened road, and the pedestrian way restored by sticking a sort of metal and plank scaffolding structure on the sides. It was perfectly safe and had been there at least ten years, but Jill had never dared to cross it.

That bridge had blighted her entire life. As a schoolgirl, she had to cross it to get to school. Rather than face it, she had played truant on so many occasions that she had, to quote her own words, 'finished up ignorant'. She could only cross it in a car, and she had worried about it to such an extent that she had made herself a nervous wreck.

Her father had brought her to the surgery in his car, for this, her seventh session of treatment. The usual arrangement was that she would telephone for him to come and fetch her, after the session. Tonight I had given her the suggestion that there was no need to 'phone her father; she could walk home, and then 'phone me to let me know that she had arrived.

Still that telephone did not ring.

*   *   *

Jill was the first person to whom I had offered hypnotic treatment, as proper therapy, but she was far from the first person that I had ever hypnotised.

The first had been a young probationer nurse, when I was a very new and brash medical student. We had been at a party, and for our age and experience had had far too much to drink. It was a nurses' party, and they were celebrating the last night of their night duty. They were all very tired, and this particular girl was feeling worse than most. Somehow the subject had got round to hypnotism, and how it could keep them going in the party spirit. All I knew about it then was some vague notion that if the subject kept her eyes fixed on a spot on the ceiling, she could be talked into it by a monotonous, repetitive voice.

Unfortunately, I made the mistake of saying so. My friends conspired, as a huge joke, to convince the girls that I really could do it, and I was challenged to demonstrate.

I knew nothing about hypnotism. They all gathered round in expectation, and my sole concern was somehow to try and save face. Through the mists of alcohol clouding my thinking processes, there seemed only one course of action: to put her in a comfortable chair, turn the lights down low and hope that as she stared at the ceiling, my monotonous voice, combined with her lack of sleep, would have the desired outcome.

With a bit of luck, sleep would come naturally and I could claim the credit for it.

It did not happen that way at all. With ferocious intensity, she stared at the ceiling, and her eyes showed no sign of closing, in spite of my ever more urgent pleas that her eyes were becoming so tired and heavy, and that she was becoming more and more drowsy and dreamy, more and more tired and pleasantly sleepy.

Some of the audience seemed to be dropping off, but not she. With fixed eyes, she stared at the ceiling. I was becoming desperate. Somewhere in the back of my mind, I vaguely recalled some film in which the hypnotist, at this point, had picked up his subject's arm and said, 'When I drop your arm into your lap, as it falls, so you will fall into

43

a deep, deep sleep.'

I had not believed it at that time, and had indeed laughed out loud, but could think of nothing else to do now.

Picking up her arm, I commanded with as much authority as I could muster, as it fell from my hand, 'Go to sleep.'

The effect was instantaneous, and incredible. She did.

The whole room stared, open-mouthed. I was terrified, I did not know what I had done. Sobering up fast, I murmured into her sleeping ear that when she woke up, she would feel wonderful. Not knowing what else to do, I told the gawping spectators that we would leave her asleep for the rest of the party, and wake her up when it was time to go home.

It somehow killed the party stone dead. They all began to leave in droves, and after a few moments there were only a few people left. With as much nonchalance as I could muster, I ambled over to her chair and said, as I gave her a good dig in the ribs, 'It's OK, you can wake up now. The party's over.'

Nothing happened. She remained resolutely fast asleep. I shook her, I prodded her, I shouted at her, all to no avail. I thought of calling a proper doctor and taking her into the hospital. We thought of taking her back to the nurses' home, but we had no transport, and students were not, definitely not, allowed in the nurses' home, particularly when carrying an apparently unconscious nurse home from a party.

Someone suggested that he shout 'Fire!' in a loud voice, and that we all rush out of the room. We did, and walked sheepishly back in when it had absolutely no effect.

In the end, the owners of the flat where the party had taken place offered to accommodate her sleeping form for the night in one of their beds; still in her party dress, she was laid in it and the blankets pulled over her.

I slept on the floor, with a cushion and an overcoat. About every half hour, I left my cold, cramped place on the floor and tried to waken her. Throughout all this, she slept blissfully on.

The dawn rose. I drew the curtains and the sunshine lit up her face. She had an expression of extreme content-ment, and I was becoming more and more alarmed and guilty. Cursing myself for my stupidity and now suffering from a quite definite hangover, I mentally went round all the different departments in the hospital, trying to decide which one to contact, and what on earth I should say to them. I had finally decided that the only correct thing to do would be to send for an ambulance to take her to casualty, and let the experts decide, when, for the first time that night, she rolled over in bed and pulled the blankets up about her shoulders.

I rushed over to her and, trying to use the same mono-tonous voice that had put her into this trance, instead of a desperate shout, said into her ear, 'You've had a lovely night's sleep. When you wake up you'll feel wonderful. As I count, you are waking up. One, two, three. Wake up!'

She rolled sleepily over onto her back, opened her eyes and gazed dreamily up at me. She reached out her arms, wrapped them languorously round my neck and pulled me down towards her. Passionately she kissed me. 'You are wonderful,' she said, 'that was the finest night of my life,' and began to kiss me amorously and urgently all over again.

Rapidly, I extricated myself and fled.

It took me six months to persuade her that I was a rotten cad, unworthy of her affection. Six months of purgatory, of hiding, and avoiding all social contact with the nursing profession.

I thought, too, that I had been put off anything remotely connected with hypnotism for life. And now, here I was again, sweating and worrying over what I had done.

The telephone still had not rung.

My watch said that eleven minutes had now elapsed. A minute is a long time, when you are waiting. I continued waiting.

*   *   *

The next time that I did anything hypnotic was quite casual

45

and unexpected, and completely unintentional. It was not just one incident, but a series.

For several years now, I had been clinical assistant to the obstetric department at the hospital. It was only a very small department, served by a visiting consultant who came in every day, but who found that all the emergencies at night were beyond his single-handed capacity. As I had once thought of taking up this speciality, and had partially trained for it, I had found that, soon after my arrival, I had been delegated to act as his assistant for three nights a week.

The salary was not excessive, but I found the work emotionally satisfying. It was all emergencies, and all at night. Since the whole unit consisted of a total of only six beds, the vast majority of babies were born at home, and only those mothers who actually, or potentially, got into trouble, were admitted.

A typical emergency admission that I had to deal with was someone who had been in labour at home for some time, and who then needed help, often in a great hurry. Naturally, most of them were extremely apprehensive, and a few quite terrified. Although, in theory, an anaesthetist was available, in most of the cases the very nature of the emergency dictated that speed was imperative, and there was not enough time to call him out and set up his gear. The whole procedure had to be done under a local anaesthetic and, in most cases, for the baby's sake, in a hurry.

A terrified, tense woman, fighting every inch of the way, made it all doubly difficult.

Over the years, I had developed a technique for calming them down and getting them to co-operate, that made life so much easier, and the delivery of a distressed baby so much quicker. It consisted, in essence, of oozing a calm capability, a calmness and capability that I rarely felt in the small hours of the morning, combined with getting them to relax, as I examined them and assessed the situation.

The relaxation was a standard set of breathing exercises, common to any do-it-yourself book on home confinements, transcendental meditation, yoga, or any other brand of eastern mysticism.

As they performed the exercises and I injected the local anaesthetic, I kept up a steady patter of soothing reassurance, and could feel the tense muscles relaxing under my fingers as I worked.

I thought nothing of it; it was just part of the preparation, like washing my hands and filling the syringe. I had never noticed that the nursing staff always left me alone with the patient while I was doing it, until one particular occasion, when a new midwife was on duty.

'Would you pass the instruments over now,' I said to her quite routinely. When they did not materialise, I glanced over to her, to see why not.

She was standing in the middle of the room, fast asleep, with a bowl of boiling water in her hands.

I was informed, after the delivery, that my relaxation patter had the same effect on the whole nursing staff, which was why they avoided me while I was doing it.

This unnerved me for a while, and I found, now that I was self-conscious about it, that it was not nearly so effective in calming down the anxious patients. It took me a considerable time and a lot of effort to regain the technique. Each time that I did it, it caused me so much worry over what I was really doing, that often I could not sleep for the rest of the night. But there was no doubt that it worked, turning many a probable caesarian section into a relatively easy vaginal delivery.

I had worried about it for a long time, as I was worrying now. That 'phone still had not rung. Twelve minutes had elapsed. I resolved to give her a few more minutes, and then I would go out looking for her, starting at that bridge.

*   *   *

Some months before, out of the blue, the morning post had brought a circular letter, inviting me to apply for a place on a medical hypnotism course. It extolled the virtues of the technique as a therapy for most of this world's ills, and stressed that the expenses of the course would be tax deductible.

Not daring to tell Mac where I was actually going, I had arranged for the time off and attended the weekend course. To my intense surprise, I found myself with a whole lot of other doctors with very similar problems to my own.

The instructors made me realise just how bumbling and ineffective I really was, and showed what could be achieved. One of the pupils, a disbelieving cynic who had only come to satisfy his own ego and show them all that it was really a load of nonsense, kept interrupting the first lecture with loud ribald comments from the back of the room.

He was courteously invited to come to the front and sit by the lecturer. From my position, also at the back, I could not hear what was said, but in about thirty seconds his eyes were closed, and he sat mute and apparently asleep for the rest of the lecture.

He sat there for the next two lectures, quite comfortably, still with his eyes closed, and for the coffee break as well. He did not leave his chair for lunch either, and was still there for the afternoon session.

When the day's session was over, the lecturer told him very quietly that he could wake up now and would remember every word that he had heard during the day. During dinner, and for the rest of the evening, he was his normal self, and when we discreetly questioned him, gave no indication that anything untoward had occurred.

At the end of the course, I bought several of the books of instruction offered for sale, and with a book in one hand and a willing patient in the other, I set about curing Jill of her phobias.

I practised on her induction and deepening techniques. One of the latter produces controlled muscle spasm in various limbs, so that they become totally rigid and unbendable.

At this stage, I told Mac all about it. He was the original disbelieving cynic.

'Can you induce total body rigidity, like the stage performers do?' he asked challengingly. 'You know, put her head on one chair, her feet on another, and then sit on her middle.'

'Of course,' I replied nonchalantly and untruthfully. His disbelief was a little irritating.

'Good,' he chortled, 'I'd like to see that. When's the next session?'

My big mouth had got me into it again. With considerable trepidation, I asked Jill if we could do this, and demonstrate it to Mac at the next session.

'I'd like to show him,' was her emphatic reply. 'He never did anything but laugh about me and that bridge.'

She was as good as her word. Mac had come to the session this very evening and had sat silent and unobtrusive in the corner, while we went through the ritual of induction and deepening. At the appropriate moment, I asked him to help me lift her off the couch and suspend her rigid form between the two chairs.

Hypnotised or no, she was as stiff as the board she was presuming to be. Mac's face was a picture as he stood back and stared at her.

'Can't believe it,' he muttered several times.

'Sit on her, then,' I suggested, not really believing it myself, and hoping that Jill would not object.

Very tentatively, he lowered himself down, expecting her to collapse under him at any moment. Jill never even sagged. With incredulity written all over his face, he lifted first one foot from the floor, and then the other.

'Good God!' He stood up, turned and stared at her. 'I'd never have believed it. What on earth have you done to her?'

'I honestly don't know,' I replied, as we replaced her on the couch.

Up to this moment, I had not given her any suggestions about the bridge, but as she had responded so well to suggestions of stiffening, I thought now was as good a time as any to do it.

I read her the standard ego boost out of the book, and then went on to tell her that it was just an ordinary old bridge, like any other, that thousands of people crossed daily without thinking about it, and that she was just one of these ordinary people.

Purely as a spur-of-the-moment afterthought, I added the suggestion about walking home, before waking her up.

She sat up on the couch and looked challengingly at Mac. 'Well,' she said, 'how did I do?'

'Incredible,' he muttered. 'Incredible.' And, picking up his hat and coat, he went home.

Jill never mentioned the bridge, or the phone call. 'I'll be off now, too,' she said. 'Thanks,' and was gone.

That was now fifteen minutes ago, and she still had not telephoned. Not only was it vital for her safety that she should arrive home without harm, it was vital that she came to work in the morning. She was our daily help, and tomorrow was the long-awaited moving day. The least I could expect was excommunication, if I had put the daily help out of action at such a time.

The telephone rang. It made me jump. 'Hallo,' I said into it anxiously, hoping that it would be Jill.

It was. A stream of abuse poured out of it. She was so angry that she was almost incoherent.

'Are you all right?' I managed to get in eventually. 'Are you at home?'

'Of course I'm damned well at home. Where did you think I was? I've had to have a hot bath and get out of these b.... wet clothes. You're going to buy me a new dress and pay for another hair-do.'

I had never thought to check on the weather before sending her home. Especially in Mac's honour, she had put on her best dress and had a very expensive hair-do. By the time she had walked home in the pouring rain both were ruined, and she was mad, hopping mad, and had no compunction about telling me so.

'I'll see you in the morning,' she threatened, and slammed the 'phone down. Not once had she mentioned the bridge. It no longer bothered her; it was just another road bridge, like any other.

6

Although a very big day to us, from the patients' point of view our moving day was a day, just like any other. It made me realise how much our own personal worries take precedence over everything else. Moving was on my mind, but quite certainly not on theirs.

They had come to the surgery not to hear about my problems of domestic disruption, but to tell me their troubles and, more important, get relief from them. The fact that I was trying to move house at the same time was singularly irrelevant. I had heard many of them all too often before and, try as I might, I could not speed up, nor stop, the full flow of well-rehearsed symptomatology.

There is a certain Murphy's Law about surgeries. When you have all the time in the world and are full of good humour, ready and willing for a pleasant social hour or so, all the patients are either in a hurry to get down to the chemist before he closes, or feel too miserable to chat. However, when, as today, there is an overwhelming sense of urgency to get done and on to the more important things, that is when people decide that now is the moment to unburden their souls and tell you all about problems that have been worrying them for years.

As usual, Mrs Pilkington had come to ease her mind. She was oblivious of the furniture van parked at the front, and the passage of heavy feet bearing our worldly goods out through the open door. She was also blissfully unaware of how impossible it was for me to take the day off, so that I had to cope with the patients and the telephone while my poor wife dealt with the packing and the workmen. My mind was not really concentrating on her ailments, real or imagined.

She suffered from her nerves, a condition brought on, according to her, by her unhappy childhood, and fixed forever by a most unfortunate event that had taken place in this very room, at the very desk I was even now sitting at. I had heard it many times before, but despite my best endeavours to hurry her along, she was determined to refresh my memory.

One of my predecessors, some twenty years before, had been patiently listening to her tale of woe and her catalogue of life's injustices, when he had suddenly, and without any prior warning, dropped dead at his desk, from a massive heart attack.

Mrs Pilkington, as she had related to me many times and was now determined to do again, had thought that it was rather rude of him to go to sleep so blatantly when she was telling him what she thought was the important part. She had merely continued her story, in a somewhat louder voice. Only a good hour later, when he had not even woken up to answer the telephone, did she think to get help. It was not the fact that the poor man was dead that upset her, it was the fact that she now had to start all over again with a new doctor who did not know her, and that she had to exist, doctorless, for nearly two whole weeks before the new one came. Fearful lest it should happen again, she insisted that every consultation should start with the distress that she had been made to suffer.

Perhaps, subconsciously, she had seen all the activity, and was determined to get her consultation in before I, too, disappeared from her life. She never once asked about the move, and I could not get a word in edgeways to tell her.

Eventually I managed to shepherd her to the door, still talking, and clutching her usual repeat prescription for nerve medicine.

She was followed by a long succession of people, all of whom were totally unaware of my other plans for the day. A few were curious and asked what was happening, but the vast majority demonstrated no interest whatever, or if they did, felt it would be rude to express it and made no comment.

Every doctor dreads the phrase, 'While I'm here, would you just look at . . .', usually after clothes have been replaced, and during the walk to the door. So often it indicates that all that has gone before was a mere preliminary to what is to follow. They were too shy, scared, or apprehensive to open the batting with it, so to speak.

The very last patient of the morning session was another of the ilk of Mrs Pilkington, inadequately equipped to cope with the modern world but who, with the aid of a veritable pharmacopoeia of pills, managed to enjoy poor health.

I resolved to restock her pharmacy in as short a period of time as possible, and get down to the serious business of moving house. Incredibly, it went very smoothly. With her prescription tucked neatly into her purse, and the latter stowed properly in her hand-bag, she had actually buttoned up her coat and was half-way to the door, when she uttered the dreaded phrase, 'While I'm here, Doctor . . .'

Wearily, I resumed my seat. The urge to show her to the door and tell her to come back another time was very great, but some sixth sense told me to be patient. Her problem might just be more important than my need to supervise the removal men.

It was. Feeling very guilty, and slightly ashamed of myself, I listened to her hesitant confession that she had a very personal problem which she had come to the surgery many times to tell me about, but had never quite had the courage and had gone off with yet another repeat of all those pills that she felt she would not need, if only she could talk to someone.

'I know it's cancer,' she said finally, 'and you can't do anything.'

On examination, her very personal problem turned out to be a copious and highly irritant vaginal discharge, with massive excoriation of the skin over most of her trunk, up to and including the area under her breasts and arms. It must have been unbearably sore and painful for months, and yet she had been too shy and embarrassed to show me before. I felt mean and ashamed of my cavalier attitude to what had obviously now been the preamble to her main complaint.

It was not cancer, it was the typical thrush infection of an undiagnosed elderly diabetic.

53

Very chastened, I sent her through the heaped furniture in the hall to the cloakroom, to produce the necessary specimen. As expected, it was loaded with sugar.

When I explained what the trouble was, she broke down and cried, making me feel even worse.

'It's not cancer, then,' she said through the tears of relief, repeating herself several times as I retrieved the old prescription and replaced it with something much more suitable and effective, together with a simple diet sheet.

'Can I stop all those other horrid pills?' she asked, as I showed her to the door for the second time that morning. 'I can tell you now, I don't think they were doing any good at all.'

'Yes,' I replied, feeling very small. Somehow the job of moving was back in its proper perspective. Next time Mrs Pilkington called, I resolved to undress her and examine her thoroughly. She, too, might just have something genuine underneath it all.

I walked through to the back, to the kitchen, in need of coffee. There was none. I was just in time to see an enormous tea chest totter by, with the kettle and coffee balanced precariously on top of the rest of our kitchen equipment, supported by a moving pair of legs.

'Mornin', Doc,' said a cheerful voice from behind it, as it passed. The voice sounded familiar, but I could not put a name to it, and could not see its face. 'How was Auntie? Came to see you this morning, didn't she?' it continued, as it passed by me into the hall.

I did not reply. Auntie could have been any one of a dozen I had seen that morning, but he did not return to repeat his question.

With the van loaded and gone, we walked round what had been our home for the last few years. It all looked so bare and desolate. We were not leaving it totally, however, for the practice had to continue from somewhere, while we searched for a plot of land on which to build the new surgery. We had arranged to rent out the upper floors and keep on the existing waiting room and surgery. The telephone engineers had installed a gadget that switched all incoming calls to our new house. Ceremonially, we switched it on and locked the doors. The receptionist and I would return to do the evening surgery.

Ruth and the children set off after the van, and I went off to do the few visits that were deemed essential.

Coming up the drive to our new manor house, it seemed so big. Not just the palatial grounds, but the sheer size of the house itself. The furniture pantechnicon, when parked outside the surgery, had seemed enormous. Here it was dwarfed by the front door alone. Walking into the front hall was even worse. When I had last seen it, it had been full of beautiful antique furniture, massive creations of oak and mahogany lining the walls. Now that they were gone, our few bits and pieces looked exactly what they were, the first few purchases of an impecunious pair of newly-weds. They sat in that great hall, looking very shabby and ill at ease.

At the time of the acquisition of most of our furniture, my salary had barely paid the rent. It had been bought, a bit at a time, with cremation fees. We had been extremely fortunate, as far as our finances were concerned, in working in a town that not only possessed a brand new modern hospital, with excellent facilities for looking after the aged and terminally ill, but also a brand new modern crematorium.

The head porter of the hospital, with the skill and demeanour of a kindly undertaker, saw to the visiting relatives. He somehow persuaded them that cremation was the only fitting end. He made all the arrangements, and we junior doctors signed the certificates. The fee for such a certificate was two guineas and, by hallowed tradition, he kept the shillings and passed on only the pounds. Those pounds, carefully saved, had bought all our furniture, at a time when we would otherwise have had to continue using orange boxes.

Now, that furniture was as out of place as orange boxes would have been and, in terms of real money, we were as broke as we had been then. True, my income was vastly increased, but virtually all of that was committed to the necessary mortgages and insurance policies. Cremation fees here were few and far between; I should have to find another source of supplementary income.

Each one of those cremation forms that I had signed contained a statutory declaration that I had no pecuniary interest in the death of the person concerned. As I had signed them, conscience told me that I was committing perjury, for I needed the fee for doing it.

While I was thinking about it, and persuading myself that I had no more pecuniary interest in such matters than the undertaker who arranged the cremation, our bedroom wardrobe passed by.

'Which room do you want this in?' said that unplaced familiar voice, from behind it. 'Auntie OK?'

At that moment a very chilly silence, accompanied by an extremely frosty look, assailed me. The frosty look was surmounted by an incredible afro-style hair-do. Jill was quite definitely not speaking to me today. She had come straight to the new house, to get it cleaned up before the furniture arrived, and had apparently still been so angry over her ruined, very expensive perm, that she had gone through the house like a dose of salts, wielding her broom and vacuum cleaner with positive venom.

I did feel a sneaking sympathy for her. Every hair on her head stuck out at right angles from her scalp, each one coiled independently like a drunken bedspring. She had tried, but failed, to hold the lot down with a brightly coloured headscarf.

''Allo, Jill,' said that voice. 'What the 'ell have you done to your 'air?'

'Ask him,' she snapped, pointing at me, and stomped off up the stairs, followed by the wardrobe.

For the first time, I saw the owner of the voice, and realised why I had been thinking about undertakers and cremations. His previous occupation had been to drive the undertaker's van. Out of context as a furniture remover, I had not recognised him.

He was an irrepressible little man, with an infectious sense of humour, who could never take any occupation seriously for more than a few weeks. He had tried many trades and had had even more employers. During one of his many spells at the labour exchange, he had amused himself by taking a correspondence course in embalming, and on the strength of this he had sought, and got, employment as the undertaker's chief assistant. It was in that capacity that I had first met him.

*　*　*

I had been ill in bed with 'flu, and feeling very sorry for myself. No patient could possibly have felt worse than I did. For the first two days of the illness, I had continued working, dragging myself round the practice with a martyred expression on my face. The last patient that I had called on, before taking to my bed and wishing to die myself, had been a very old lady clinging to life with a grim tenacity, whose departure had been expected hourly for weeks.

She passed away peacefully during the night, and I signed her death certificate from my sick bed. This I could do without seeing the body, but to issue a cremation certificate, I had to examine it.

The undertaker's chief assistant arranged the cremation to his entire satisfaction, but could not proceed without my certificate. Having been firmly and politely told that I was not leaving my bed for anybody, dead or alive, he announced that he had no alternative but to bring her to me.

Mac was taking some of my surgeries and, being so taciturn himself, had not exactly encouraged enquiries about my health. All that the patients knew was that I was ill in bed, and had not been seen for a week.

Whistling a happy little tune, the chief assistant walked in through the front door, followed by four men carrying the coffin. They put it down on the hall floor, and the only open door being that to the waiting room, asked the assembled patients for instructions as to where to go.

Hearing the noise, Mac left the consulting room and, positively hissing in anger, instructed them in vernacular Scottish to take it round to the back door. Still whistling cheerfully, they obeyed.

Speculation in the waiting room, we learned afterwards,

was rife. They all knew that the coffin was for me, but, as was pointed out with conviction, it was too small for me. Likewise, it was too big for any of the children. The only one it could possibly fit was my wife, and they had all seen her that morning. Mac did not enlighten them.

Sweaty, faint and horrible, I crept down the stairs to the back porch, where an extremely irate wife had refused them further entry.

Here, I certified, with shaky hand and sweaty palm prints, that she was indeed dead, had no bullet holes or stab wounds, and could safely be legally cremated.

*   *   *

Shifting furniture was a much more suitable occupation for the cheery little man. Now that I had recognised him, I also knew who his auntie was. She was the lady whose diabetes I had missed for so long.

He and Jill came down the stairs together for the next load.

'Been meaning to have a word with you about Auntie,' he said, interrupting his happy whistling for a moment, and grinning wickedly at Jill's new hairstyle. 'She's a poor old thing, you know.'

'I know,' I said, involuntarily grinning back at him as, with her nose in the air, her hair flying behind her, and a very haughty expression on her face, Jill walked by, cutting me dead. 'I think we've got to the bottom of it at last. We'll soon have her right.'

By the end of the day everything was in place, the men had been well tipped, and Jill had been partially mollified by sufficient funds to have her hair redone. At least she was speaking to me.

We walked slowly round our new home, savouring every moment. The rooms that had not looked so big when full of the previous owner's massive furniture, looked cavernous with ours. The wallpaper, that had been unobtrusive before, glared bare and hideous from the great exposed open spaces.

We stood in the hall. 'Are you aware that you can count

seventeen different clashing wallpapers from here?' Ruth asked.

'Does that matter?' I countered. I was watching the children racing up and down the hall, chasing each other with shrieks of delight. The first part of the dream was coming true; details like changing the wallpaper could come later.

'Can we have our bath in the swimming pool?' they were demanding. 'Please,' they repeated, jumping up and down in excitement.

It was only when we were in the water that we discovered that it stained us all green.

7

It was a glorious summer. We worked and worked in the garden, and still could not see any progress. The lake was our pride and joy.

The only trouble was that the lake was inhabited by a swarm of nondescript geese, and a vast army of muscovy ducks. These had reduced the vegetation to a sea of mud, apart from the odd patch of stinging nettles, so that there was no natural food for them at all. They were entirely dependent on the food that we took down to them twice a day, and this they ate in prodigious quantities.

Individual muscovy ducks have been made into pets on many occasions, but none of these could be classed in that category. The drakes were great, ugly black and white things, with a head full of red wattles, whose only function seemed to be that of hissing at me when I went to feed them. They stood on the same spot of land by the food trough, waiting all day for more, and fouling it ever deeper with their droppings. The only time that they moved at all was in order to drive off a duck that tried to get a mouthful out of the trough. The ducks did have some endearing qualities, like huddling together on another part of the island, looking very pathetic. At first the children loved to feed them for me, but they totally failed to make any rapport with any of the birds, and invariably came back stinking of duck muck. The excuse, from whoever was asked to feed them, that he was still in his school clothes or just going out somewhere, came to be repeated thrice nightly, as we did the rounds of the children. Establishing a rota of duty caused more family rows that it saved arguments.

We had promised the previous owners that we would look after the birds, but this was too much. The weekly food bill was horrendous, and no matter how much we gave them, they seemed to demand more, and more, and more.

Throughout that first autumn and winter we carried food down to the island in ever increasing quantities. Even the wild mallard, hearing of our bounty on the duck grape vine, came to feed, in their thousands it seemed.

The mud got deeper and deeper, and so did we—into debt, paying for the food.

Slowly, imperceptibly, came the first signs of spring. It was no longer dark setting off to the evening surgery, and daffodils started poking their noses through the sea of mud. Not a blade of grass grew down there, and most of the daffodils were soon trampled on by the geese, as they rushed up and down fighting each other for territory.

At last, we thought, eggs. We should be able to sell most of them to recoup our losses. Shelters were built of straw bales, and straw nests made everywhere. The geese just marched up and down the lot, treading it into the mud. Every day, we took down more straw, and hunted in vain for the first egg among the wreckage of yesterday's nests. When we did find it, it was in the water. Just lying there, all wet and horrible, and very muddy. No one fancied eating it at all. Sporadically others appeared, in the most unlikely places, but seldom in the nests that we had so laboriously built.

The moment of truth arrived: selling them. We couldn't even give them away, not even to our best friends. We tried to eat some ourselves, not enjoying them at all. Andrew, now nearly six, expressed the family feelings when he was forced to eat one boiled for his tea. He shovelled it in, with silent protest written all over his face, and then threw up all over the table. Duck eggs were not served again.

A great load were sent to the local market. The goose eggs fetched a few shillings, but the muscovy eggs, so diligently washed by hand to make them more attractive, came to less than the auctioneer's minimum commission. The local carrier's bill came to exactly one shilling more than the money from the market.

We lost interest in picking up the eggs and left the birds to their own devices. In no time at all ducks and geese were sitting on eggs everywhere. They still demanded the same quantities of food, however.

The broody birds settled down to wait the statutory incubation period for the chicks to hatch—thirty days for the geese, and thirty-five for the muscovy ducks. Naturally, the children wanted to know why the birds were spending so much time asleep, sitting on the eggs, and dozens of questions arose, such as why they did not break the eggs when they sat on them. We used this time to very good advantage, and tried to answer their questions by explaining the facts of life.

John, being the eldest, at seven, stood on his full dignity and outshouted his younger brothers, being quite convinced that they had misunderstood the whole process. They resolved to settle the argument one morning at breakfast, with the telephone going full blast, from patients who could not wait till the morning surgery, and amid frantic preparations to get everyone off to school in time.

'You do lay eggs, don't you, Mummy?' he said.

George, being deemed by his elder brothers to be very ignorant by the fact that he was only four, burst into tears as he ate his scrambled egg and refused to touch any more, until he had been completely reassured that he was not eating his baby brother.

He spent the rest of the day loving the Harry cat very passionately, not really convinced by the explanations of viviparous birth, given in haste between mouthfuls of toast and marmalade. The Harry cat was a stray that had just walked in one day, made itself comfortable in front of the stove in the kitchen, and by its actions declared itself fully at home. We called it the scraggy cat. It was thin, moth-eaten in appearance, and jet black. It was a long-haired cat, and where the hair was particularly long, these hairs were of a brownish colour. The children called it Harry, familiarised to the Harry cat. In return for food and shelter, it suffered the most outrageous indignities, constantly being clutched to one bosom or other, and carried about the house at all kinds of angles and postures. It was dressed in dolls' clothes, pushed about in the pram and, to our eyes, horribly maltreated, but it seemed to love it, keeping up the loudest purr of any cat I have ever heard. Being named Harry, we all came to assume that it was of the male sex, and nobody ever bothered to check. About the time that the geese started sitting, however, the cat started to get fatter round the middle. At first we assumed that this was just due to good feeding, but with suspicions aroused, it was subjected to a sex test and pronounced, without any shadow of doubt, to be female. Despite this, it remained the Harry cat.

Naturally, we used this new-found knowledge to illustrate further the parable of the birds and bees, watching Harry's tummy growing bigger. There was a daily ritual laying on of hands, to see if we could feel the kittens moving inside. When, after about two weeks, nothing had happened, the children became impatient, expressing serious doubts not only about their father's powers of diagnosis but about the whole theory of procreation as well. The race was on. Who would hatch first, a duck, a goose, or the Harry cat?

Harry won by one day. Things had been imminent all that day, and she had been very restless and unsettled. All during their tea, round the kitchen table, Harry had been mewing in discomfort, wandering from corner to corner of the room. We put a cardboard box, lined with a piece of old blanket, in front of the stove, and Harry leaped in and settled down, apparently going to sleep. Tea over, the children all went up for their communal bath, hurried through it and came down in their dressing-gowns full of excitement, to watch the first kitten being born. Their little faces were full of wonder and astonishment, not so much at the performance of the cat, which was exactly as described, but at the fact that Dad had been proved correct.

Four kittens were eventually deposited in front of the stove. Naturally, one each. Every one was distinctly different—one tabby, one black, one ginger, and one black and white. In order of seniority, each child claimed its newly born kitten. It would have been a major calamity if there had been only three, as little Elizabeth, the only girl and the youngest at three, would have been considered by her brothers too young actually to own a cat. She, however, was in fact the boss, getting her own way by dint of sheer volume of noise whenever she was thwarted. The boys always gave in to her desires. She was the one who did most of the loving of the Harry cat. Gripped tightly by the neck in both her hot little hands, she carried it everywhere. At times we feared that she might strangle it, but the cat did not appear to mind and just kept on purring. Never once did Harry even offer to scratch her in return. It would have been unthinkable for her not to have a kitten all her own. With great difficulty she was persuaded not to take one to bed with her, but to leave them all with their mother in the box.

Next morning, when we came down to breakfast, the children had obviously been up for hours. In an endeavour to give the cat some milk, they had managed to spill the last two bottles all over the floor, breaking one of them. There was no milk for early morning tea, let alone breakfast, and worse, even though they had managed to clear up most of the mess, there were still small pieces of glass all over the floor.

They predicted, quite correctly, that I would not be pleased, and lined themselves up in a row for chastisement. The boys saw the inevitable logic of crime and punishment, and prepared themselves manfully for it. Not Elizabeth. Quite oblivious of the reason for my anger— mainly no cup of tea—she put down the kitten she had been cuddling, reached up her little arms, and said with the full force of female charm, 'Poor Daddy's cross. Let me kiss him better.' Totally devastating.

John, however, had thought of something even better to distract me. 'Dad,' he said at just the right psychological moment, 'if you look out of the window, one of the ducks is up on the lawn with fourteen baby ducklings.'

Spilt milk forgotten, we all rushed out to see them.

A muscovy duck with ducklings is a transformed being. It looked pleased with itself, and very proud and maternal. Anatomically, there is no way that a duck can indicate a facial expression, but somehow they do. This one looked so satisfied and fulfilled. As soon as it saw us, it called all the ducklings to it with a purring throaty rattle, and

64

advanced, completely sure that we represented food. It was not wrong, and the children had a marvellous time trying to persuade the ducklings to eat out of their hands. All too soon, it was time for work and school. The boys and I went off, leaving little Elizabeth proudly in charge of both her new families.

During the ensuing weeks, dozens of broods of ducklings hatched out. None, of course, had the same emotional impact on the family as the first one. There were just too many, and four tiny kittens that could be played with, fed and loved, were much more entertaining than ducks. We were glad that this was so, as we really thought that all these ducklings represented saleable duck meat, return on the hard-earned money that had been guzzled throughout the previous year. But no matter how many fresh broods hatched, there never seemed to be any more ducklings on the island. They were disappearing at roughly the same rate as they hatched. John was the first to notice why.

'Dad,' he said one evening, 'I think that the drakes are drowning all the ducklings. They chase them around till they catch one, and then hold it under water, and it doesn't seem to come up again.'

On my next day off, I made a special point of going down to the island, to spend an hour or so watching the drakes. John was quite right. Usually, the only time I spent watching them was at feeding time, when all they were concerned with was eating. Once the trough was empty, they set about the ducklings. Drifting apparently aimlessly about the water, any duckling that came within their range was seized and held under water. Since most of their activities took place at the water's edge, the little bodies were soon trodden into the mud and disappeared.

Those drakes had to go. The local butcher would have to be contacted, or rather nobbled when he next came into the surgery. I thought he owed me a favour. He had put his fingers in his mincing machine again, making it the third time that I had had to stitch them up in recent months. He always made his sausages first thing in the morning, and as he started work at four a.m., mending his fingers was done in the middle of my night.

The fourth occasion occurred sooner than expected, when a telephone call again woke me up at that ungodly hour and was greeted with the usual flood of obscenity as I composed myself to answer it.

'Ronnie here,' said the telephone, even before I had managed to speak into it. 'I've done it again, Doc. Can I meet you in the surgery in ten minutes? Good, I'll see you there,' and he rang off. One of these days, I thought he is going to get a wrong number and frighten some poor old lady to death; or perhaps better still, he will ring the police station, and get booked for abuse of the telephone. Wearily I dressed, deciding to wash and shave later, just in case he bled to death on the surgery steps—or more accurately, if I was not there within the ten minutes, he would only ring again.

I met him at the back door of the surgery and we went into our special little treatment room. I was very proud of this room. We had all the facilities for doing minor surgery, dressings and so on, keeping all the instruments sterile and ready in covered trays of spirit, just for occasions like this.

He had made a proper job of his fingers this time. Three of them were in shreds. I was seriously doubting my competence to have a go at reassembling them as I sat him down and put his hand on our very new, very expensive surgical table. I expressed my doubts to him, but said that I would clean up the wounds, and then decide if he would need specialist care in suturing tendons and so on. Ronnie had no such doubts. I had made the same speech last time, then with courage in both hands and heart in my mouth, had sewn up a single tendon on the back of his little finger. Mercifully, it had healed beautifully, and his finger was fully functional.

To give myself time to think, I shoved a thermometer in his mouth, so that he would not talk and break my concentration; then I began to wash the wounds in disinfectant solution, assessing the extent and nature of the injuries as I did so. It was not as bad as I had first feared, and I thought that I could do it.

I took the thermometer out of his mouth—his temperature was of course normal—and told him what I thought.

'Good,' he said. 'Every time I have to go down to the hospital, it's the best part of a day waiting around to get served. If I treated my customers like that I should soon lose the lot.'

While we were talking, I injected some local anaesthetic into his hand. I used what is known as a ring block, injecting the anaesthetic in a ring round the base of each finger, in order to block the nerve to the finger and so totally numb it.

'Ronnie,' I said, 'this is the fourth time this year that you've mangled your fingers in that sausage machine of yours. How have you managed to do it four times?'

He thought for a moment before he answered. 'Just carelessness, I suppose.' And after a pause, 'No, not carelessness. Trying to get the job done faster. You see, we cut up all the meat that's to go into the sausages into rough chunks, and put it into the hopper over the mincer. The original hopper didn't hold enough, so we built a big extension over it, that would hold all the meat to be minced for the day. If some of the chunks are too big, they form a bridge across the mouth of the mincer, so that the machine keeps on running but nothing goes through it. Every time I pass the mincer, I give the meat a shove down, to stop it bridging. Sometimes it needs a good hard shove, and if it suddenly gives, whoops, watch your fingers.'

'Can't you use a stick or something?' I said.

'Yes,' he said, 'but then I get splinters in the sausages, and the public health boys are on my back.'

'You'd better get a new machine,' I told him, 'because next time you won't have any fingers left.'

I checked that his fingers were numb and then began the long job of stitching them up, one finger at a time. I did the worst one first. Fortunately the bones and joints appeared intact, but the tendons on the backs of the fingers were severed, and the palmar surfaces badly bruised and torn.

'In return for services rendered,' I told him, 'you are going to buy some ducks.'

'Not those damned old muscovies on your pond, I'm

67

not,' he said.

I stitched away with a minute needle and nylon thread at the tendons on the backs of his fingers. It was quite a tricky job lining up the tendons exactly, and snipping off the jagged edges so that the two cut surfaces joined exactly and were held in place by the nylon sutures. Nylon had to be used as tendons take so long to heal, and something more or less permanent is needed that will not be absorbed before union is complete.

Having joined the tendon, I then started to restore the fine sheath enclosing the tendon, ensuring that the tendon could move freely within it and that my nylon knots did not catch on it. For this I used very fine absorbable catgut that would be completely dissolved and gone in a few weeks.

I moved on to the relatively easy part, using the usual black silk for the skin.

'About those muscovies,' I said, and told him of the problem of the drakes killing all the ducklings.

'Only natural,' he said. 'Too many birds in too small a space, Mother Nature's birth control. I can take the young ones, if they've any meat on them, but those old drakes, no.' He shook his head vigorously, moving his hand on the table.

'Keep that hand still,' I reminded him. 'I can't hit a moving target. Surely you can do something with them, even if it's only putting them in your sausages.'

'No, Doc, not even for you would I put them in my sausages. They're much too old and too tough.' He wriggled a little as I stitched. The local anaesthetic was wearing off, so I put another shot into the last finger. 'Someone gave me a goose for Christmas during the war, that wasn't nearly as old as your muscovies. I had one hell of a job to kill it.' He screwed up his face at the memory of the struggle to break that neck. 'Well, eventually I got it dead, plucked and dressed it, and gave it to the wife to cook. She's a good cook, my wife, and she roasted it, and we invited all the family round for Christmas dinner.' He shifted in the chair, gesticulating as if to indicate the size of his family.

'For goodness sake,' I almost shouted at him, 'keep still.'

His unexpected arm waving had made me jab the needle into my own finger.

'That goose,' he continued, quite unperturbed, 'was so tough I couldn't even cut a slice off it. I hacked and sawed and sharpened my knife again, and I couldn't even dent the skin. I had to nip over to the shop and get some sausages, and we had them instead. Some Christmas dinner! The wife took it back into the kitchen and steamed it all afternoon, and I still couldn't cut a slice off for supper. She steamed it all that night, and I tried again on Boxing Day, and still could not cut it. We threw it in the dustbin in the end—even the dog couldn't chew it.'

'Yes,' I said, 'but that was a goose. These are ducks.' 'No difference,' he interrupted, 'and the flesh will taste of old marsh mud. Tell you what I'll do, as soon as this hand of mine is mended, I'll bring some chaps over and we'll catch the lot, and take them over to a mate of mine to put into his game pies.' I smiled with relief. 'He owes me, time I collected!'

'Thank you,' I said.

'Mind you, only when my hand is better. I'd enjoy a bit of sport duck catching.'

I finished off the suturing, covered all the wounds with antibiotic powder, and then gave him a tetanus injection in his other arm.

'You might have put that in the same arm,' he grumbled. 'Now I shall have both of them out of action.' I took no notice, pointing out that he was lucky that penicillin now came in capsules he could swallow. He would certainly need some antibiotic, and injections of those were very painful. If he did not stop grumbling and promise faithfully to dispose of all those muscovies, I would arrange for the district nurse to call and give him a daily injection.

'I promise,' he said. 'The boys and I will be round on Sunday morning, and we'll take all the drakes we can catch. And,' he added as an afterthought, 'we'll come and get the rest as soon as they're big enough.'

Thus was the fate of the drakes decided. He was as good as his word, and they were duly rounded up and dispatched. We all resolved not to eat any game pies for a

69

while, and felt very sorry for those who would pay good money for them. Whatever Ronnie got he kept, for I never received any money for them, and did not have the nerve to ask him for any when he returned to the surgery to have the stitches removed. Rather to my surprise, but to his intense satisfaction, his fingers healed up beautifully, with no trace of infection.

*   *   *

Life was not all roses after the departure of the drakes. Not one goose had hatched anything, despite the fact that the books said that they had a shorter incubation period than the muscovy ducks. All the incubating geese just sat there, ever hopeful, but nothing happened. One by one they gave up, and abandoned their nests. We opened one or two of the unhatched eggs, to find that they contained nothing but an evil-smelling liquid. Whatever life they might have had in them once had long since died and putrefied.

The last remaining goose continued to sit, with a seemingly feverish desperation to resurrect the life within the eggs. The more time that went by, the harder that goose sat. She had been sitting for about six weeks, when John and I were pottering about down on the island one evening, and both jumped into the air as a loud bang just behind us really startled us. It was exactly like a gun going off. We turned round, and there was the sitting goose standing up over the nest, with an expression of intense distaste on its face, as it peered underneath it, watching a thick custard-like material drip down from its chest and outstretched wings. One of its rotten eggs had exploded underneath it. It rose from the nest and, with its wings outstretched, tiptoed with immense dignity down to the water. Its whole body expressed horror and disgust as it waded in and, when the water was up to its knees, performed a series of bobbing up-and-down manoeuvres, in a futile attempt to wash off the mess. From where we were standing, several yards away, the smell was extremely horrible, and from where the goose stood it must have been unbearable, representing, as it did, the end of dreams of motherhood.

All the other geese came rushing up and stood in a line on the bank, facing the unfortunate bird, and with their wings held well out, and their necks stretched as far as they would go towards her, honked with derision or sympathy—we could not tell which, but they were certainly expressing some emotion.

The remaining ducklings were not doing well, either. They seemed to thrive for about two weeks and then go very thin, getting weaker and weaker until they died. We feared that they were not getting enough food and gave them ever more, but it made not the slightest difference: a few more died each day. On the principle that one body is much like another, and that the medical training I had so rigorously undergone had well grounded me in pathology, I thought that a quick *post mortem* examination of a corpse should reveal the cause of death. Such an examination was duly performed, but all it revealed was that I knew nothing of the internal anatomy of a duck, and if there was disease there, I did not know what to look for. After about twenty-four hours, the insides had decomposed to a uniform greenish-black mass of tubes that bore no relation to anything remotely resembling the insides of a human.

The whole family had gathered round the kitchen table to watch the operation, each one convinced that father had the power and magic of Dr Kildare and, with a shout of 'Eureka!', would discover the cause and remedy it. I might just as well have opened the entrails to predict the future as to do a *post mortem*; both were equally obscure. However, I had to keep my reputation intact, so pronounced that there was nothing obvious and it must be an infection, and that we would need proper culture done by the local vet to identify the organism responsible. This seemed to satisfy the children, but Ruth gave me one of those looks that wives give their husbands when they catch them out but do not wish to puncture their ego.

'What we shall do,' I said, 'is go down to the island first thing in the morning, catch one of the sick ducklings and

71

take it down to the vet, to see if he can make it better.'

This was duly agreed. One was caught and Ruth took it to the vet's surgery.

'I felt such a fool,' she told me later that night. 'I sat in that waiting room for nearly two hours, holding that duckling, surrounded by people with cats and dogs. I got some very funny looks.'

Eventually she was ushered into the consulting room, and laid the now expiring duckling on the table.

'That duck's dying.' the vet said.

'I know it's dying,' my wife replied. 'That's why I've brought it to you, to find out why.' And she explained how the others were dying in droves, and how unsuccessful I had been with a none-too-fresh corpse. The vet agreed to send it off to the nearest veterinary investigation centre for proper cultures to be done, quickly put the poor little thing out of its misery, and popped it into a polythene bag.

About a week later we received the report. It was accompanied by the bill from the veterinary investigation centre for five pounds, and another from the vet for two more. The report stated, 'This bird died from a broken neck. It is very thin. There are no other obvious signs of disease.'

It was, I suppose, a very effective way of getting rid of bothersome people. I wished that I could dispose of some of my bothersome patients just like that. We took the hint and did not trouble them again. They were, after all, specialists in animals, not ducks, and probably knew no more than I did.

When the few survivors were big enough, I rang Ronnie and he came and made a grand clear-out of everything—to make more game pies, I supposed. Again, he never raised the question of payment and neither did I. After all, the birds had been caught and taken away. The lake and island seemed terribly empty and almost haunted by their ghosts, but at least the haemorrhage from our bank account had stopped. It had been an expensive year, but we felt very guilty and missed them more than we had ever anticipated. Even the kittens, which by now were half-grown cats, did not seem to compensate, and the children, who had done the most grumbling about the work involved, missed their daily trip with the food buckets.

It is said that out of the mouths of babes and sucklings comes forth wisdom. George, who had said nothing but had obviously been deeply affected by the manner of departure of the birds, came and sat on my knee one evening, snuggled right up to me and whispered, 'Dad, could we get some pretty ducks, so that when we sell them they won't have to be killed to go away? And we only sell them to people who want ducks to look at, not ducks to eat.' Not only could I have kissed him, I did.

But where to get some pretty ducks? We should have to find out.

8

'It's not fair,' I said as I came in from my afternoon's visits and saw the packed mass of humanity sitting in the waiting room. I was quite sure that I felt much more ill than any of them. My head throbbed, my nose was blocked, and my chest was wheezy and sore.

Outside the temperature was still well below freezing, with a thick fog that was thinning to a mushy rain, rain that turned to ice as it hit yesterday's snow still lying on the pavement.

'It's not fair,' I repeated to my wife as we huddled over the fire having a quick mouthful of tea before I started the evening surgery. I was late and it was going to be another of those horrible nights. Prior to the National Health Service, my medical predecessors had welcomed such packed surgeries. They had called it the harvest season. Mac and I called it sheep dipping. Mac had developed the technique to perfection.

'Time and motion,' he said, when I asked him how he managed to get through five patients to my one. 'You don't need to drink the whole pot of soup to know what it tastes like.'

I must have looked suitably blank.

'Consider it logically,' he continued. 'The patient comes in, sits down and tells you that he's got a cold. You know he's got a cold, and whatever his chest sounds like, you're going to give him a prescription for some antibiotics and cough linctus.'

'I hadn't thought of it like that,' I replied dubiously.

'Well, think about it now,' he told me. 'Every one of them has an overcoat on, and underneath that, a jacket, a cardigan, a shirt and a vest. It takes three minutes to take that lot off, and three minutes to put it all back on.'

I nodded my agreement. Some of my old ladies took ten or fifteen minutes each way to unpeel and replace their

74

multitudinous garments.

'Now,' he said, 'you've got thirty people waiting out there. Thirty multiplied by six minutes is three hours. They don't want to waste three hours, and neither do you.'

I hesitated to tell him, but I could not get through that lot in less than four.

'All you do is undo the top button of their shirts and insert your stethoscope under the vest. One quick sample breath to the left, one to the right, and give them the prescription.'

'But that's a travesty of an examination,' I protested.

'So it is,' Mac replied, 'but it's all ninety-nine per cent of them need. You cover yourself by telling them that if they are not better by the time they have finished the course of antibiotics, to come and see you again. Any that return, you give the full works to, including an X-ray and blood count.'

In spite of myself, I had found that I was following his advice. On evenings such as tonight, I could dip sheep faster than he could.

I was tired. It had been one hell of a day. Unsolved problems crowded in on my mind. I began to dip my sheep, hating myself for practising medicine in such a superficial and uncaring manner. A sort of rhythm developed. The patient sat down, told me his cold was now on his chest and, before he could say anything further, my stethoscope was inside his shirt, first to the left, then to the right, and before he could protest, he found himself on the doorstep, clutching a prescription for antibiotics and decongestant cough linctus, while I ushered in the next sheep to dip.

Every so often a patient who had not got a cough sat down in the chair. Half of me welcomed the challenge of something different, the other half resented the interruption to my high-speed rhythm.

Skin rashes, indigestion, vaginal discharges, they all went through the dip at high speed. On nights such as these, I relied heavily on intuition. Mac and I had often talked about it.

'I don't know how, and I don't know why,' he told me, when I confessed to him my fears of missing something

75

important during such mad-rush surgeries, 'but I have already decided whether I am going to strip and examine a patient before he or she has even sat down and started to speak.'

I, too, had found that I was developing his seat-of-the-pants medicine.

Enid Wilson walked in and sat down. 'I've had a filthy cold for a fortnight,' she said, 'and it's really settled on my chest.'

My stethoscope hung limply round my neck, and stayed there. I sat and waited for her to continue. I knew her vaguely. She had never married, but stayed at home to look after her ailing mother and non-coping father. Her father had died some years previously, but her mother had enjoyed ill health until a ripe old age. She had been a demanding and querulous old lady, subtly blackmailing her daughter with the unspoken threat of dying alone and unloved, should she ever be left on her own.

Up until her death, a few months ago, I had called regularly on the old lady to restock her chemist's shop of pills. Enid, although always present, had kept very much in the background. Even in the last few weeks, when I had called almost daily, I had never got to know her, our conversations always being about her mother. I had never examined her, and her medical record cards were virtually blank. Enid had not been permitted to be ill.

'I seem to have been so run down since Mother died,' she said slowly. 'Every cold and sore throat that's about, I seem to catch.'

I looked at her closely as she talked. Her overcoat was soaking wet, and from underneath her wet, nondescript hat a few straggly grey hairs poked out. She looked much older than her forty-two years, and the make-up and rouge on her face failed to disguise her pallor and ill health.

'My ankles are swelling a bit, too,' she added, and when I still did not say anything, she continued all in a rush, 'I really didn't ought to have bothered you, when you're so busy, but my ... friend,' groping for a word that would not tell me that her friend was male, 'insisted that I come. I'm sorry. I'll come back another day, when you're not so busy.'

She stood up and turned to the door.

'Sit down.' She sat down, looking flustered and embarrassed. 'Take that wet hat and coat off, I want to have a proper look at you in a minute.'

She took them off. Her dress hung untidily about her. She had obviously lost a lot of weight recently.

'Have you any pain?' I asked her gently.

'Only the usual,' she replied, somewhat surprised, 'but it has been a bit worse recently.'

'And where's that?'

'Here,' she said, rubbing the right-hand side of her tummy. 'I've had it so long, I've got used to it.'

'Any difference in your bowel habits? Diarrhoea or constipation?'

'No difference, but I've had diarrhoea for years, that's normal for me.'

'Any blood in it?'

'Oh, yes, but only a little.'

Inwardly I groaned. It was ominous. I knew just what I would find when I examined her. At my request, she undressed and lay on the couch. The whole of her abdomen was full of craggy, cancerous lumps. It had also spread to her lungs. The swelling of the feet was secondary to a failing liver, replaced by cancerous growth. She had but weeks to live.

'How long have you had this pain and bleeding?' I asked as I felt her tummy.

'Oh, several years. It's been going on so long, I didn't think it mattered.'

'Whyever didn't you come and see me about it before?'

'Roger wanted me to, Roger's my friend, by the way.' She paused, as guilty as a twelve-year-old schoolgirl caught snogging behind the bicycle sheds. 'But I couldn't, not with Mother being so ill. It didn't get any worse, so I didn't bother.'

'Is this Roger serious?'

'It was once, but Mother didn't like him. She wouldn't let him come to the house.' She paused, and looked appealingly at me. 'He's only a carpenter, you see. He

77

worked for Daddy.'

'But you've been friends all these years?'

'Yes,' she replied shyly. 'We're going to get married in the spring. We're just waiting till a decent interval after mother's death.'

'Put your clothes back on,' I told her, and walked back to my desk.

She dressed and sat down. 'Could you give me a tonic, some vitamins or something, to buck me up a bit?' she pleaded. 'It doesn't seem right. Roger and I have been waiting fifteen years to get married, and now it's in sight, I'm just too tired. Do you think a vitamin tonic would help?'

'Yes,' I lied, and wrote a prescription for morphia and cocaine elixir. 'This will make you feel better.'

'It's not fair,' I thought, as I showed her to the consulting room door. I walked down the passage with her and opened the front door.

'Thank you,' she said, 'and good night. Would you like me to send you an invitation to the wedding?'

'Please,' I replied. She walked out into the night, her shoulders hunched against the rain, and her coat wrapped around her.

'There's no justice,' I thought, 'it's not fair.'

I walked back into my consulting room. The next patient, a big, fat domineering woman, was already seated in the chair. She looked over her shoulder at me as I entered the room, glaring her disapproval.

'It's not fair,' she complained. 'I was in front of that other woman, and she's kept me waiting twenty minutes. It's not fair.'

'No,' I agreed with her, 'it's not fair,' and resumed dipping sheep.

9

To a dairy farmer, birth is a natural and a necessary thing.
If his cows do not have a calf each year, they do not give
milk. It is as simple and as natural as that.

It was just as simple and natural that when William took
a little time off from his cows to marry his girl from the
farm next door, she should have his son the following
spring.

The problem was that it had not happened. His girl,
Dillys, was one of those rare creatures, a natural beauty,
with an inner grace to match. If she entered a room, most
of the males in it automatically stood taller and adjusted
their ties. They never stood a chance. Since her early teens
she had only had eyes for William, and he worshipped the
ground she stood on.

She had first come to see me when she was barely sixteen, and asked if she could have the pill. I was impressed
by her poise and maturity and, had I not married one very
like her myself, I should have been very envious of young
William.

I had asked her the usual questions and checked her
blood pressure which, like the rest of her, was absolutely
normal. Physically there was no reason why she should
not have the pill, but I was more than a little apprehensive
about giving it to girls of sixteen.

'Does your mother know that you've come to see me
about it?' I asked her, 'and if I give it to you, will she come
after me with a meat hatchet?'

'No,' she said hesitantly, 'she doesn't know. I think she
would be a bit upset, but you won't tell her, will you?'

'No, of course not,' I reassured her. 'But you see, you
have put me in rather a delicate position. If you are already
sleeping with him and have come to me for protection, of
course you can have the pill, but if you are thinking about
it, and my giving you the pill means you will say "yes"

79

when you should have said "no", Mother will have good reason for coming after me with the meat hatchet, won't she?'

She had smiled that inner knowing smile, that made her look extremely beautiful, and which informed me that what she did with William was their own personal secret. The radiance that it gave her told me clearly that she was already a fulfilled woman and no longer a little girl.

I had prescribed the pill.

My non-medical friends have often asked me what I feel, performing intimate examinations on so many nubile young women, so often, as a part of my job. The honest answer, in the vast majority of cases, is nothing.

Learning to do it, as a student, was an entirely different matter. I have memories that I would rather forget of the acute embarrassment that it caused both parties.

Mac explained it once to an avid audience. 'It's like this,' he said. 'When I am examining an ankle, one ankle is much like another ankle. I know what should be there, I am not admiring the shape of it, I am looking to see if that shape is distorted from the normal, if it is swollen or bent. I am looking for bruising or redness. I feel for tender spots, and I check that it moves in the normal manner. Emotions are not involved, the whole thing is cold and clinical.

'It is exactly the same with any other part of the body. One woman looks much like any other woman on the examination couch. You know exactly what they've got, and under the antiseptic conditions of the examination, it arouses no feelings whatsoever.

'It isn't what a woman's got that excites a man, it's what she does with it.'

I agreed totally with Mac's assessment. For the vast majority, he was perfectly correct, but there is always the odd one who is magnetically different.

Dillys was such a one. As far as I was concerned, she knew what to do with it. But then, she had that effect on every male within a hundred yards of her, and was deliciously unconscious of it. The only man that would ever enter her life was William, the boy from the farm next door.

80

Every six months she came to see me for her pill check, and I watched her blossom and mature. They had sent me an invitation to the wedding, but I had been unable to go.

And now, one year after their marriage, they had both come to the surgery, very bashful, to ask for help. She had thrown her pills away on their wedding night and, to their great amazement, nothing had happened; she had not conceived.

I examined both of them and ascertained that they were both exceedingly healthy; then I delicately enquired whether they were actually doing the right thing. I presumed that a dairy farmer would know just what it was all about, but I remembered only too well a couple in my student days, who had been fully and intensively investigated for their infertility before it was discovered that he was trying to inseminate her umbilicus. She had volunteered that they found sex unexciting, and occasionally painful.

It was always as well to check the obvious.

The next thing to check would be their lifestyle. A very busy life of long hours of hard work can in some instances inhibit ovulation, especially if it is accompanied by a great deal of stress and worry. They looked a little askance as I asked them about this, so I told them Mac's favourite infertility story. It concerned a couple, patients of his who had been married for seventeen years. They earned a living as market gardeners, working extremely hard all the year to produce the fruit and vegetables that they sold on their stalls in the various towns in the area. They had done a full day's work by the time most people rose from their beds, and then spent the rest of the day selling it from their stall. No family had appeared, so they just kept on working, and they had never had the time to see a doctor about it. Nor, throughout this time, had they ever had a holiday. This particular year, after seventeen years of working seven days a week, every week of the year, they had decided to take a holiday, and gone to Skegness for a fortnight. To their utter amazement she had become pregnant and was so delighted with the outcome that they had made it an annual pilgrimage, and in no time at all had acquired a

81

large family.

'So you see,' I told them, 'it is relevant to enquire about the stresses and pressures in your life, and the other ridiculous thing I must ask about is close-fitting underpants.'

They both looked at me in disbelief, and Dillys began to giggle.

'No, I'm serious,' I said. 'All male animals hang their testicles outside their bodies, not so that you farmers can castrate them more easily, but to keep them cool.'

Dillys's giggling became uncontrollable, and William started to blush. 'Mother Nature,' I said, trying hard not to laugh myself, 'has proved that in order to produce adequate sperm, the testicles need to be several degrees cooler than the rest of the body. If man in his wisdom chooses to hold them back up again, they can become overheated and fail to produce viable sperm. You can achieve the same thing with too many hot baths,' I added, and William blushed ever deeper. He obviously did wear tight underpants, and had a scalding hot bath every night to remove the smell of cows.

'The next thing to do,' I told them when they had recovered, 'is to find out whether you, William, are producing viable sperm, and you, Dillys, are actually ovulating.'

I filled in the form for the sperm count and handed it to him. 'The path lab will tell you how and when to produce the specimen,' I told him.

He regarded the form with distaste. 'I always felt sorry for the bulls in the AI centre, having to perform into an artificial cow,' he said, 'but I never thought that I should have to do it myself.'

I shared his revulsion. I do not think I could have done it in cold blood, either, but then, I was not desperate to find out if I could father children, I already knew. Stopping any more coming was my problem. As usual, I chickened out of the technical details, leaving it all to the pathology lab technician to explain the gruesome procedure.

'Now, Dillys,' I said, 'your turn. Luckily for you, there is a nice simple way to find out if you are ovulating each month. I'm going to lend you my special thermometer. It's just the same as an ordinary one, but the spaces between the marks are much wider, so that it is more accurate. You take your temperature every morning, before you get up, and, of course, before that first cup of tea, and record it on this special chart. Ovulation normally occurs fourteen days before the next period, and if it occurs, you will notice a slight rise in your morning temperature at that time.'

I handed her the thermometer and the blank chart.

'Keep it up for three months,' I told her, 'and if it shows that you are ovulating but haven't conceived, then we can go on to the next stage, to find out if your tubes are open.'

'It's much easier with cows,' William remarked as they stood up to go. 'You can tell when they are on heat. The trouble with women is that they are on the whole time.' Dillys punched him gently in the chest as she blushed delightfully, and then pushed him towards the door.

'Lucky you,' I said to him, as they went out. 'But don't forget to save your strength for the morning that her temperature rises.'

It seemed no time at all before she was back in the surgery. I knew she was pregnant as she walked in. She had that radiant look, with the characteristic softness round the eyes, and a blooming translucency of the skin.

'I'm only a fortnight late,' she said, 'but I feel a bit sick at times, and I'm sure I am. I just know it in my bones.'

'Good,' I replied, 'I'm sure you are, too, but it's far too early to examine you. Go away and be normal, and we'll start all the antenatal nonsense when you've missed your second period.'

'Thank you,' she said, 'I was hoping you'd say that, but it's really William I've come about. He's gone all bashful about that sperm test and won't go and have it done. He gets all embarrassed when I mention it. If I am pregnant, does he really need to go through with it now?'

'Good heavens, no,' I replied. 'All we wanted to know was whether he was capable of being a father. If you are pregnant, we know he is, and you can tear that form up. The test won't tell us anything we don't know already.'

She handed me back the fertility thermometer and the chart, still blank. I looked at it. 'You didn't use this either, then,' I said.

'No, but thank you for giving it to me, and for being so understanding with William. He hated coming, you know, and it took me about six weeks of nagging to get him here. As soon as we got home that night, he took all his under-pants out to the cowshed, as washing cloths for the cows' udders, and the next morning he booked us into a hotel in Skegness for a fortnight. I didn't use the thermometer, as I forgot to pack it.'

'There's something about that Skegness air,' I told her. 'Two of ours were conceived there. Don't do what we did, and go every year, will you?'

'No,' she said, 'one at a time.'

*   *   *

Her pregnancy was utterly uneventful, and she sailed through it.

As soon as he realised that she might be pregnant, William treated her more like a queen than ever. She was not allowed to do anything, and more or less banned from the farm, where she had been working quite hard.

By the time that she was really beginning to show her condition, she admitted to me, at one of her routine monthly checks, that she missed all the work and wanted something to look after, but could think of nothing that did not involve work, that William would approve of.

'What about a tank of tropical fish?' I joked. Old Herbert Allcock was now up and about again, and had come to the surgery on his old resurrected motor bike. It had taken longer to mend than he had done.

'What a good idea,' she said, 'I'll go and see him on the way home.'

On reflection, after she had gone, I did not think it was such a good idea. It had only been a joke, but it could well backfire if she started humping buckets of water about for the aquarium.

When she came the next month, her conversation was nothing but fish. She told me how Herbert had come out to the farm, sized up their sitting-room and fitted them a tank into an alcove. He had set it all up, filled it with plants, and a week later brought the fish.

'It's absolutely beautiful,' she enthused. 'We watch it in preference to the television.'

'I know,' I replied, 'he set up one for us once. I used to watch it for hours. All that activity going on in total silence, that's what I liked.'

'I can't keep my mother away from it,' she laughed. 'She insists on feeding them every few minutes, and she gives them far too much. You must come over and see it some time.'

'Yes, I will,' I said, 'when I'm passing by, and I've got a few moments to spare.'

I was passing by a few weeks later, and on the spur of the moment called to see the fish. The aquarium was, as she had said, strikingly attractive. We talked of fish, and of cows, and I told them my saga of the muscovy ducks, and of how I now wanted some ornamental ducks but could not find any for sale. As I was about to take my leave, Herbert's battered old motor bike came carefully up the farm drive. He, too, had called to check on the fish.

With ponderous delicacy he negotiated the furniture to the fish tank, and peered into it from very close up.

'You are still giving them too much food,' he pronounced. 'If you keep on at this rate, you'll turn the water grey and poison everything, fish, plants and all.'

'It's Mother,' said Dillys apologetically. 'I can't stop her feeding them.'

'You'll have to,' he replied. 'Hide the food, then she can't give it to them.'

'Would you like a drink, you two?' William interrupted. 'The sun's over the yardarm, and I'd love one.'

'No, thank you,' replied Herbert, before I could answer. 'I never touch alcohol. I only drink that what's natural. Do nasty things to you, that stuff, can't it, Doc?'

'Yes,' I replied with feeling. 'And no thank you for me, too, as I must be off.'

'I'll bring you some nice plants for that lake of yours, come the autumn,' Herbert said as I was leaving. 'I've got some lovely bulrushes. If you get any more ducks, they won't eat those.'

85

'Do you want to bet?' I replied, forgetting that this, to, was decried by the brethren.

'No,' he replied solemnly, 'but they won't.'

The last few months of Dillys's pregnancy passed very quickly. About ten days before she was officially due, the midwife called me to say that she seemed to be in early labour. I went round after surgery, but by the time I got there, she had gone off the boil; it was a false alarm. We all had coffee instead. I noticed that the fish tank had lost its previous sparkle: the plants looked a little tatty round the edges, and the fish seemed heavy and sluggish, but I made no comment.

Grandmother had come up from Wales to help out over the next few weeks. After I had been introduced to her she told me that she intended to be present at the birth of every one of her great grandchildren. She had seen all her grand-children born, and she was not going to miss any of the next generation.

'Never seen anything like those fish, boy,' she said. 'Fascinating, aren't they?' and she poured half a packet of food into the tank. 'I must go and see how my marmalade is getting on,' and she walked off into the kitchen.

Dillys opened the tank, and tried to get most of the food out before it sank. 'She's a dear, but I'm going to have to hide this food again.'

A lovely smell of boiling marmalade came from the kitchen, as Grandma lifted the lid off an enormous saucepan to stir the contents.

'She believes that she'll always be welcome if she keeps us in marmalade,' William explained. 'Every time she comes, she spends most of her time here making it. We've got enough to last us about two years already, but she does so enjoy making it.'

Two days later, Dillys had another false alarm. After I had examined her and confirmed that she was not really in labour, we had more coffee. The water in the fish tank looked distinctly 'off', and more marmalade was boiling in the kitchen.

I put the packet of fish food in my pocket and said that I would return the next day. In fact, I did not, as the midwife

86

'phoned me to say that there was nothing doing, except that Grandma had insisted on her taking half a dozen jars of marmalade home with her after her visit.

She 'phoned me again on the afternoon of the following day, to say that Dillys was now definitely in labour. I went round after evening surgery to assess progress. Things were moving. Nature was taking its course.

I examined her. Everything was normal, but it would be an hour or two before the baby was born, and it was hardly worth while going home as she was getting on so fast. I decided to wait there, rather than run to and fro.

As I came down the stairs, the smell of marmalade rose to meet me. Grandma was at it again, but this time the smell was not inviting. There was an aroma of something rotting, of marsh mud and corruption, that became stronger as I advanced down the hall.

I went into the sitting-room, and here the smell was overpowering. It came from the fish tank. The water was grey, foul and opaque. All the fish were lying on the surface, desperately gulping air. Another half-empty packet of fish food stood on the top. Emergency action was needed, to change the water before all the fish died.

William was working somewhere down on the farm, and Mother had temporarily disappeared. There was only Grandma busy at her marmalade in the kitchen—and me. I had a little time to kill, so I thought I might just as well clean the fish tank as sit and suffer the smell.

I went into the kitchen and asked Grandma for a couple of buckets and, if possible, a bit of hose pipe, to act as a syphon. She produced them with a puzzled look, and it never crossed my mind to tell her that I wanted them to clean out the fish. A few minutes later I returned with both buckets full of evil-smelling grey fluid which I tipped down the sink, and asked for some hot water. Grandma never said a word.

I made a second trip. This time the grey fluid was even more evil-smelling, and when tipped down the sink completely overpowered the aroma of marmalade.

I refilled my buckets with fresh water and took the kettle into the sitting-room, to warm the water up to aquarium temperature before I tipped it in. On my return to the kitchen for more boiling water and another two buckets of cold, Mother had reappeared and, as I walked out with them, I heard Grandma whisper hoarsely to her, in the broadest Welsh accent, 'Good God, girl Gladys, whatever is he doing to our Dillys?'

Having poured the water into the fish tank, I was about to go back to the kitchen and explain when the midwife called down the stairs, asking me to go straight up. I went up at a run and arrived in time to witness the most natural birth of the bonny boy everybody wanted. My presence was not really necessary, as everything was so normal.

When it was all over, I left the midwife to clear up and went downstairs to tell the family. William had returned from the farm and all three were standing in the kitchen, white-faced and scared, with the evil smell of the fish tank still lingering to add credence to the tales of horror with which he had been regaled.

It was with the greatest of relief that they learned that I had only been cleaning out the fish tank while I waited for Dillys to get on with it.

'You've got a splendid son,' I told William, 'and they're both fine. You can go up and see them in half a moment, as soon as the midwife has finished making them both look beautiful, and on the way up, you can pour us all that drink we didn't have the other night. I think we could all do with it.'

Stiff whisky in hand, we all trooped up the stairs to drink the baby's health and tell Dillys how her fish had been rescued.

Grandma presented me with a dozen jars of marmalade.

*   *   *

I called in every day for the next few days, just to ensure that all was well. Mother and baby thrived and really did not need my services, but it was such a pleasure to see them all so happy that I called anyway.

Grandma was very contrite over her excessive feeding of the fish—perhaps I really called to medicate them. All bar one survived the experience, but the plants did not respond to treatment. After full consultation, it was decided that we would have to bring in the specialist.

'Unfortunately,' said Herbert, when I called to see him and explained the catastrophe, 'the old bike is not blessed with the healing powers of the flesh. The main frame has broken.'

I took the hint and arranged to take him over there one evening the following week, with a tankful of fresh plants.

While Herbert was planting up the tank again, William and I sat on the sofa talking.

'You remember you told me you wanted some ornamental ducks?' he said. 'Well, look at this,' and he passed me the local paper. At the bottom of one of the middle pages was a short article saying that a bird garden on the North Norfolk coast was closing, as the site was to become a housing estate. Its entire stock of birds would shortly be coming up for sale. 'I've got to go up that way on Wednesday, to take some calves I've sold. I'll be going up in the lorry, and I know Wednesday is your day off. Would you like to come up with me?'

'Well, yes, thank you.' He had taken me completely by surprise.

'I've jumped the gun a bit,' he continued, and my face must have been a picture. 'I 'phoned them up, made an appointment and gave them the impression you might take the lot.'

When I finally got home that night I was bubbling with it, and rushed in to tell Ruth all about it. Unfortunately, I had stayed gossiping far too late, and she was in bed, fast asleep. She was so used to my comings and goings in the night that my arrival did not wake her. This worked the other way round with the children. If one of them needed attention in the night, she would get up to deal with it, not waking me.

I told her all about it at breakfast next morning.

'You know we can't afford anything like that,' she said, 'so don't go and do anything stupid. How much do these birds cost each, anyway?'

'I don't know,' I replied, 'but it will be fun finding out.'

On the Wednesday, William called for me, with his lorry

89

full of calves. We delivered them and then went on to the bird garden. There seemed to be an awful lot of ducks there, of all shapes, sizes and colours. I was absolutely fascinated. Ruth had brought me a book on ducks from the library, and we walked round trying to identify the various species, without much success.

The owner came over to join us. 'I've got a list of everything here,' he said, and handed me a sheet of paper. It was the price list of a duck dealer, on which he had marked the numbers of each of the many species that he had. I noticed that many of them were only single birds, not pairs, and the prices were marked by the dealer in many pounds each.

Desperately trying to think of a way in which I could get out of buying anything, without telling him that I could not possibly spend so much money on ducks, I said, 'But I'm only interested in the breeding pairs.'

'That's no problem,' he replied, pointing to the dealer's list. 'You can get anything you want from him. He'll make up the pairs for you. I've marked it all down, what sex they are.'

It was a good job he had, because I could not tell one from another, but I dared not say so.

William came to the rescue. 'What are you asking for them? Not that full list price?'

'No,' he said, 'the usual: two thirds, if I have to catch only a few. I tell you what I'll do. I want to be rid of them as soon as I can. If you take the lot, you can have them for half.'

William, on my behalf, and probably because the day was fading fast and he wanted to get back home to his family, said, 'Done. Let's start catching them. What have you got to put them in?'

I stood there open-mouthed as dozens of orange boxes were produced and, with a fisherman's landing net, the ducks were unceremoniously scooped up, boxed and loaded into the lorry. My mind refused to function as I tried to calculate how much it was going to cost. Several times I opened my mouth to shout, 'Stop! Let them go, I can't pay!' But I did not say it. I wanted those ducks.

90

Whichever of the ten commandments it was that started, 'Thou shalt not covet thy neighbour's goods', I was breaking it; I coveted his ducks. It was a blessing we had a friendly bank manager, for, although he did not know it yet, he was going to lend me the money, and how it was to be paid back would be his worry.

In no time at all, the ducks were loaded and the calculations done. They came to a frightening sum of money, even at half price. I wrote out the cheque and signed it, praying that I should be able to persuade the bank manager not to bounce it.

Just as we were about to go, the bird garden owner said, 'Hang on a minute, I've got a whole load of bantams, sitting boxes and coops and runs. Are you interested?'

Before I could open my mouth to say 'No! I've already spent more than enough for one day,' William had answered, 'Yes, but a few old bantams and second-hand runs aren't worth much. We'll take them off your hands as discount.'

To my complete amazement, I heard the reply, 'Go on, then, bring your lorry round the back and pick 'em up.'

There were not just a few, there were masses. Before I lost count I had registered sixty bantams and a dozen cockerels, and we had quite a performance getting all the coops and runs onto the lorry.

'Thank you,' I said to William as we drove away, 'I couldn't have done that.' And as an afterthought: 'I haven't got any food. Where on earth am I going to get enough for all that lot?'

'No problem,' he replied. 'We'll call at my place on the way, and I'll lend you a sack or two till you can get some delivered.'

When we arrived home the whole family came out to see us unload the lorry. 'What on earth have you got there?' Ruth asked, consternation written all over her face.

I handed her an orange box full of bantams. 'The complete do-it-yourself kit of duck breeding,' I told her. 'All we need now are a few odd birds from the duck dealer, to make up the breeding pairs,' and I passed her the price list.

'However much have you spent?' but before she could

say any more William rescued me again. 'He's had a damned good deal,' he said. 'He's bought all the ducks for half price, with the hens and the equipment thrown in for nothing. It was an offer he couldn't refuse.'

We let all the ducks out of their boxes on to the lake. They looked magnificent. 'What sort is that one?' Ruth asked.

'It's a Chiloe Widgeon,' I told her proudly, 'but she needs a mate. I'll ring up the duck dealer in the morning and get one for her. If we're going into the duck breeding business, she must have one.'

'Yes,' she said dubiously, and continued looking at the ducks. 'Can we really afford all these birds?' Before I could give her an honest and considered answer, she went on, 'That little whatsit widgeon does look lonely. We'll have to get her a mate, at least.'

She walked up and down the bank, looking for more lonely hearts, apparently accepting the fact that we had acquired yet one more possession that we could not afford.

We unloaded the bantams into the old chicken run and piled all the coops, water pots, and other equipment that I had not noticed in the loading up, into a big heap. Then we gave the birds some food and went indoors to talk ducks and dream dreams.

We didn't 'phone the duck dealer the next morning, we 'phoned him that night. He was out but the voice on the other end of the line said, 'I know he'll be up your way tomorrow. I'll get him to call and see you.'

We made elaborate plans, so that Ruth would be able to contact me at any moment during the day when he came. Naturally, he never showed up. When we came to know him better, we realised that he had no sense of time. An appointment for a certain day could mean any day a fortnight either side of it. The time of day was a little more accurate, for he could never be more than twenty-four hours out.

He came, unannounced and unexpected, just as we were about to sit down to Sunday lunch. His car, a little red low-slung two-seater, was filled to capacity with boxes of ducks. He parked it just outside the back door, and from somewhere in the middle of all these boxes, a long thin figure uncoiled itself. He was well over six feet tall, and wore an old blue mackintosh that hung on his spare figure like a collapsed bell tent. The very first illustration in Ruth's library book of ducks was of an Australian Magpie Goose, perching precariously in a tree. Standing there, unloading boxes of ducks, he was the original for the illustration.

Leaving the lunch steaming on the table, I went out to him. He introduced himself diffidently and held out a limp hand, then continued unloading his ducks. It was just like a conjuring trick. The pile of boxes grew ever bigger, and there seemed to be just as many still in the car. I felt almost tempted to walk round the car, to see if someone else was loading them in from the other side; how he had got that number of boxes into such a small car intrigued me, it was not geometrically possible.

When they were all out, he said, 'I heard you'd bought the bird garden and wanted the pairs made up. I've got most of them. Shall we carry them down to the lake?' He set off, like a circus juggler, with eight of the boxes balanced one on top of the other. I followed precariously with two. The children, who had quietly left the table and formed a ring of engrossed spectators, followed with one each. He opened the boxes on the lakeside and released the occupants on to it.

Ruth came out to watch the proceedings. Her little Chiloe Widgeon came steaming up to the bewildered newly-arrived drake, chatted him up and down, and took him off to the far side of the island for the serious business of courtship to begin. We all stood there for a few moments, admiring them. 'Your lunch is on the table getting cold,' she said, and, turning to the duck dealer, 'Would you care to join us, because if it isn't eaten now, I'm going to put it in the dustbin.'

'Oh, gosh, er,' he replied. 'Is it that time already? Er, yes, thank you.'

During the course of lunch it became apparent that he knew every duck we had acquired, its age, its parentage and its potential breeding capacity. In the few short

93

minutes that he had watched our birds, he had absorbed everything.

'I haven't brought you a New Zealand Scaup,' he said, 'or a Fulvous Tree Duck Male. I should be able to get those in the next few days.'

He ate very delicately, not at all like a Magpie Goose which, I imagined from its picture, would be a greedy feeder. The children pestered him with questions; so much so that he had little time to eat, and we had all finished almost before he had started. They were silenced, and in embarrassed solitude, he picked at his dinner while they gazed at him in open admiration. He knew more than Dad about ducks and must therefore be a very special man.

After the meal, we sat over the dishes talking ducks, and before we realised it, it was tea time. Ruth cleared the dirty plates away and replaced them with clean ones.

'Why do we need all those hens?' asked John. 'Why can't they sit on their eggs themselves and hatch them?'

'That's a good question,' he said between dainty mouthfuls of cake. 'Several reasons, really. First, the duck eggs are too valuable to be left lying about down there. A rat might eat them, or a crow, or some small boy break in and steal them. Secondly, when the duck is incubating them, every time that she is disturbed off the nest, the eggs get cold. With all those birds down there, something is always disturbing them.'

He took a genteel sip of tea and wiped his mouth with his handkerchief. 'And the third and most important reason is that if you take the eggs and put them under a hen to hatch, the duck will lay a second clutch of eggs, and then possibly a third, so that you will get many more ducklings than if you left them for her to hatch.'

'Doesn't it upset them when you steal their eggs?' George chipped in.

'Oh, yes, of course,' he replied, 'but no more than if a rat ate them, or if they were knocked off their nest by a bigger duck. They soon get over it, they don't spend days grieving like people do.'

We talked of nesting boxes, we talked of broody hens, we talked of food, and at the children's bed time, we all went down to the island to feed them. The one thing we did not talk about was money.

The children were sent off to bed and we sat round the fire drinking coffee. The afternoon slipped quietly into evening, and soon it was midnight. He showed no signs of going, accepting each coffee as it was offered, and all the time we talked of nothing but ducks and the technical details of feeding them, mating them, hatching them and rearing them. At about two-thirty in the morning, it suddenly dawned on me why he was still here: he wanted paying.

With great tact, I raised the subject, starting with the enormous sum that I had paid for the first consignment from the bird garden, and how I hoped he would give me a similar discount for quantity.

'Ah, you were very lucky there,' he said. 'I called to see him just after you had left. My normal buying price is two thirds of my list price, and that's what I would have given him. Fortunately for you, I was held up.'

I stared at him in horror. At his full list price, we owed him an enormous sum of money; not even our friendly bank manager would honour a cheque for that size. We would just have to go out and catch them all again.

He was speaking, and I had missed the first part of what he was saying. 'Everything that you breed I will take from you at two thirds list price. The snag with a lot of people is that they sell off all the good stuff at my list price, and then expect me to pay two thirds for all the commoner ducks that they can't sell. If we agree that I'll buy them, I want all of them, and you don't sell another duck to anyone else.'

It seemed too good to be true, and I agreed to the proposition with alacrity.

'We, er, I will put the ones you bought today down on the account, then, and we'll deduct them from your breeding sales next year. Er, in this business, there is always next year.'

And so it was agreed, but still he did not go. Two cups of coffee later, I told him that I should have to start morning surgery soon.

'Oh, gosh, er, is it that time already? I had better go. I

should have had lunch with my sister today. I'd better go tomorrow.'

At precisely ten past four, he loaded up all his boxes and drove away. Bug-eyed, we went to bed.

*   *   *

The next weekend, William brought Dillys and the baby to see the ducks. Grandma and Herbert sat in the back of the car, holding two great plastic bags full of bulrushes. The boot was crammed full of other pond plants.

The women went into the house to talk babies, while the three of us planted Herbert's tribute. Up to our knees in water, we dibbled them into the mud. A voracious army of hungry ducks followed behind, pulling them out again— Herbert's language was unbecoming of such a devout Christian. Grandma was recruited to throw bread at them, in the hope that she could distract the ducks long enough for us to hide the plants, but although we succeeded temporarily, within a week they had found and eaten every one.

Later that evening, we stood on the bank admiring our handiwork and watching the antics of the ducks.

'I prefer them to fish,' said Grandma. 'They're sensible, I can feed them as much as I like.'

'You know, you could be on to a good thing,' mused William. 'If every duck lays ten eggs, you could get a tenfold return on your capital.'

To a stockman and farmer it was so simple and natural. In the spring, ducks lay eggs, that are reared into more ducks, that make a lot of money.

With prophetic insight I replied, 'I wish they would, but these are wild birds, you know, with at most one or two generations in captivity. They're not going to behave like your domesticated cows. If we're lucky, we'll rear one or two youngsters per pair. I doubt if we'll get as much as our money back in the first year.'

Little did I know how right I would prove to be.

96

10

Ivan the Terrible earned his living with a mechanical digger. That was not his real name, just his reputation. His parents had christened him Frederick, and until he bought his ancient digger he was known to the world as Fred Shotton.

He was a small, extremely muscular man, proud of his strength and even prouder of the fact that the huge, hydraulically rammed arms of his digger were merely an extension of himself. He handled them with an artistry that belied the brute strength behind them.

There was no hole in the ground, no matter how large or how dangerous its approaches, on whose rim he would not work happily perched; no slope up a mountain of earth too steep for him to charge. He had struck terror into the hearts of many a building site foreman by the frenzy and reckless energy with which he attacked any piece of offending earth.

The digger had at one time been the property of a firm whose name had been painted in large letters on one huge digging arm: 'THE WIVANHAM CONSTRUCTION COMPANY.'

Ivan had inadvertently burned off the initial 'W' with his welder, when mending a cracked joint, and lost everything else bar the 'IVAN' when he had broken and replaced the upper arm.

With a pot of paint, someone had crudely written ''THE TERRIBLE' on the new arm and the name had stuck, despite the fact that the paint on the arms had long since rusted off.

Ivan had supreme faith in the abilities of both himself and his digger. He knew of no hole, or situation, that he could not dig his way out of.

*   *   *

97

He stood at the bottom of the garden, pushed his cap to the back of his head and thoughtfully scratched his bald pate.

'It'll cost you, Doc,' he said.

'How much?' I asked anxiously.

His head scratched to his satisfaction, he replaced the cap.

'Don't rightly know, till I've worked it out.' He rubbed his chin while he thought. 'It'll be a fairish job. Could take a couple of weeks. I'll work it out on a bit of paper and let you know.'

Inwardly I groaned. We walked back to his car. 'See you next week,' he said as he drove off.

Disconsolately, I walked back into the house to report progress.

Like most people, having bought a house, I had blissfully assumed that when one pulled the chain and watched one's waste products disappear round the proverbial bend, that was the end of the matter. In a house not connected to the main sewer, it is not the end, but only the beginning of a very involved and complicated process.

The previous owners had just been a simple twosome who had not made great demands on the ancient system. The surveyor had looked into all the manhole covers and reported that the drains, although ancient, appeared to be working efficiently; apart from reading his report before we bought the place, we had not given them another thought, merely noting that drainage was by cesspit and soak-away.

We had to think about them now, for they were intruding into the very heart of our existence. The six of us, together with the ever-working washing machine, had filled the entire system. We were pouring it in at the top end faster than it could absorb it at the bottom.

At first the full lavatories, that emptied themselves overnight, had just been a joke, but when they failed to empty at all, the joke turned sour.

Draining rods were acquired and pushed full-length into the dark recesses, in all directions. This stirred the ancient sediments and the upper waters receded, only to return after less than a week. Our self-congratulation was short-lived.

The council offered to pump out the cesspit, and an enormous tanker duly arrived.

'Where is it?' the driver asked. We sheepishly told him we could not find it and, after searching for a whole day, he had to admit that he could not find it, either, and took his still-empty tanker away.

By measuring the length and direction of the drainage rods, and digging holes at every apparent obstruction, we located three bends in the pipe, two unsuspected manhole covers and, finally and triumphantly, the main catch-pit. It was under two feet of earth and about six more of garden compost, at the top of the yard.

Ivan was summoned, with his digger, to move the compost heap and expose an entrance. He did in one hour what would have taken me a month with a spade. Unfortunately, he lifted the concrete top off the whole structure, which guaranteed its ultimate demise.

The council tanker came twice weekly to pump it out and, intimating that this was only a temporary expedient, ordered us to replace the entire system. Connecting us to the main sewer was just not possible.

Ivan returned to give us an estimate for digging the new one. He informed us that we would need a thing called a carjester (which was apparently an enormous hollow pot buried many feet underground), several hundred yards of herring-bone pipe and numerous other things, besides the cost of two weeks of his labour putting the lot deep into the bowels of the earth.

Wearily, I sat down at the kitchen table and reached for the tea pot.

'I am fed up with blocked pipes,' I told my wife. 'Half the practice seems to have some pipe or other blocked inside them at the moment, and now if the house pipes aren't blocked inside, they're blocked in the garden.'

Silently and sympathetically, she poured my tea.

Trying to console myself, I spoke my thoughts aloud. 'I'm off duty this Sunday. I'll get the rods out again and see if I can find the outlet pipe from the catch-pit, and dig down and clear it.'

We both sat there in silence. New sewers cost money; not only had we not got any, but after the purchase of all those ducks, the stretched overdraft was pushing against even the friendly bank manager's limits.

'Never mind,' she said. 'We've been in debt before, but with a bit of luck you'll clear it before Ivan returns with his estimate.'

Sunday morning came, and very early the boys and I trooped out to see what we could do. We had barely started when Ruth came running out of the house.

'It's Peter, the policeman, on the 'phone. He says someone has buried himself in a hole, and can you get over there quick.'

Swearing, I went into the house to speak to him. I had enough troubles with holes of my own, without being bothered by other people's.

'It's Fred Shotton,' he said quickly. 'The sides of a soak-away have collapsed on him. Can you get over there quick?'

'Fred Shotton?' I said. 'I don't know him, do I? Where's he live?'

'Course you know him. Ivan the Terrible on the sides of his digger,' and he gave me quick directions to his house.

Leaving the boys to put away the barely used tools, I leaped into my car and drove to Ivan's house. I arrived on the heels of the fire brigade.

A small crowd had already gathered and were standing round the collapsed hole in his garden. Someone was running out of the house with an armful of spades. The top end of a buried ladder poked up out of one end of the hole.

'What happened?' I asked one of the bystanders, as the firemen seized the spades and, with the energy of a pack of Jack Russell terriers, began a frenzied attack on the heap of earth down in the middle of the hole.

'He was digging a new soak-away with that thing there,' nodding at the digger parked at one end of the hole. 'He'd got down to twelve feet and was still in clay. He'd gone down the hole with a spade to see how far he'd got to go till he hit the sand.' He looked at me, correctly assuming my ignorance. 'Water won't soak away through clay. Got to get down to the sand, you know.'

'And the sides fell in on him,' I said, stating the obvious.

'That's right,' said the man, walking round to the other side of the hole where he would get a better view.

I followed him round and, as we walked, the earth moved a little; for a moment, I thought that more was going to fall in and bury the firemen as well.

'Get back there,' shouted the chief fire officer. 'Get away from the sides, you bloody fools. This isn't a peep show.'

The crowd duly moved back.

I looked at the sides of the hole. It seemed to me that the lot was about to fall in at any moment. The firemen were too busy with their frenzied digging to notice. I walked over to the officer, introduced myself in my capacity as emergency doctor summoned by the police, and tentatively suggested the digging stop and the sides of the hole be shored up, before we had half a platoon of firemen buried in it.

'You're quite right,' he said as he rushed round, trying to establish some semblance of calm and order. 'I've already sent for some timber.'

'There must be some here,' I suggested. 'Some old doors, perhaps?

He came to a halt and swung round to face the crowd.

'Doors!' he shouted at them. 'Bring me all the old doors you can find!'

Given something positive to do, the crowd moved purposefully towards the house, led by a largish woman who I presumed was Ivan's wife. Within moments they had returned with what looked like the garage doors, and the front door as well. Reluctantly, the digging firemen paused in their activities long enough for the doors to be lowered down the sides of the hole and propped in place with whatever was handy.

They were only just in time. The one previously intact long face of the hole sagged against the newly installed door. Desperately, the firemen propped and levered it.

'More doors, and find some props, anything you can to hold it up!' shouted the officer. I found myself inside the

101

hole, desperately levering a garden rake against one corner of the advancing door. I eventually got it in position, each end of it bracing a door on either side of the hole. The rake handle held, but it curved up in the middle like a well-stretched bow.

The firemen paused for breath. I grabbed a spade. They had been attacking the whole great heap of caved-in earth from the top, passing each spadeful to a colleague reaching down from the rim of the hole. Thinking about it, it seemed logical that Ivan would have seen or heard the side caving in and would have run for the ladder. The most likely place to find him would therefore be near the ladder. Nobody took the spade away from me, so I began to dig methodically down.

After two spadefuls, I thought I saw a finger. Throwing the spade to one side, I knelt and reached into my little hole. Frantic scrabbling uncovered a hand. I reached in and caught hold of it, giving it a squeeze to see if there was any response.

The hand gripped my fingers so fiercely, it hurt. Instinctively, I squeezed back.

'Here!' I shouted. 'I've uncovered his hand. He's alive!'

That hand gripped mine so tightly that I could not move; I was stuck in an increasingly uncomfortable kneeling position, reaching down. Two firemen knelt down beside me, digging with their hands.

'Follow his arm down,' I gasped. 'His face will be at the end of it somewhere, and we can get some air to him.'

Frantically they dug, passing out each lump of heavy clay to willing hands behind. The hole around his arm grew deeper. A hissing air hose dropped over my shoulder from above. Not knowing what to do with it, I poked it up his sleeve. It seemed to slip in quite easily, so I pushed it up to what I guessed was one arm's length. The hand squeezed mine a little harder, in what I took to be a gesture of thanks.

From above quite large clods of earth fell on my head. Our hole filled up again. The door above me bulged ominously. I could not move; it was pressing over at an angle, against my back.

There seemed to be a hundred firemen's legs around me as they grunted, pushed and shoved. A door descended beside my head. I could only think it was the bathroom door, for it was white, and stuck on it was one of those comic transfers, of a cartoon baby on a pot, and underneath it the legend, 'The job is not completed till the paperwork is done.'

In my awkward, cramped position, it seemed that I stared at it for hours, but eventually the walls were shored up again and the firemen resumed digging. All the while the hand clung desperately to mine, and the air hose hissed up his sleeve, and the door pressed against my back.

Eventually the diggers uncovered down to the back of his neck. His head had been forced sideways and down, away from the arm that we had uncovered, and rammed forcibly into the rungs of the ladder. As the firemen moved the earth from the back of his head, I leaned forward, still holding his hand, slid the fingers of my other hand along his neck to his ear and heaving awkwardly upwards, removed a huge, heavy, wet lump of clay.

The clay was removed from my hand as soon as I had loosened it. I leaned forward to speak into the exposed ear. I wanted to use his name, but could not remember it. The only name I could remember was 'Ivan the Terrible'.

'Ivan,' I said, with as much soothing confidence as I could muster, 'we've got you now. You're OK.' I felt that my voice was shaky, and far from soothing and confident. More lumps of earth thumped on my back, and I could feel the weight of it increasing. Ivan's ear disappeared from view again several times, as the falling earth reburied him. Above and around me I could hear strains and grunts and muffled curses, as the desperate shoring-up continued.

It seemed a desperately slow process; to steady my own nerves as much as to reassure Ivan, I kept up a running commentary of what we were doing.

'Can you hang on a bit longer?' I asked him. He gripped my hand tighter in reply. 'They're having a bit of trouble shoring up the sides properly. We can't really get on till they've done it.'

Eventually we got his head clear. He had only been

103

saved from suffocation in the first fall by being at the base of the ladder. There was a small air space between it and the earth wall, into which his face had been rammed.

Quite inadvertently, I had saved his life, in the second instance, by misjudging the length of his arm. It was much shorter than I had anticipated, and I had pushed the end of the pipe right past the centre of his chest to his left shoulder, up to the point of his chin, where it had been unnaturally forced, so bringing him a new air supply as the space beneath the ladder filled up with falling earth.

He could hear us, but he could not see or speak—his eyes and mouth were too full of dirt. As I cleaned them I continued my commentary, trying to keep us both calm.

'Soon have you out of here, Ivan,' I kept telling him. 'They've just got to move the earth behind us to give us some more room.'

What I did not tell him was that there was now only room for one fireman and me down in the bottom of the hole. The top of one side had completely fallen in, pushing the shoring relentlessly towards us. The shoring on that side, I took to be a bedroom door. It had been covered, French style, in wallpaper, cream coloured, with badly drawn purple roses splattered all over it. Each time I screwed my head round to look at it, those dreadful roses seemed nearer and more menacing.

We finally got his upper shoulder as well as his head free. An urgent voice whispered in my ear, 'Can you get a rope round him, quick?' Since I last looked, those roses had advanced six inches. There was barely room for the two of us. The fireman burrowed frantically on his side to find the other arm, while I tried to make a space between Ivan's chest and the ladder. I passed the end of the rope into the hole I had made, the fireman groped and clawed along his burrow until he just managed to reach it.

Thankfully, we pulled enough rope through, and the fireman skilfully knotted it.

'We'll pull him out,' came a voice from above. 'Mind your backs. Pull!' Uselessly we attempted to help lift from the bottom, as they pulled from above.

Ivan screamed, the first sound that he had made. 'My

104

arm,' he croaked, 'it's trapped.'

'Hang on a minute!' shouted the fireman, 'I'll see if I can free his arm.'

'For God's sake hurry up,' the anxious voice came down. 'We can't hold this shoring much longer.'

The sense of urgency was affecting me. With a horrifying lurch, those roses sagged towards me. The child on his pot moved down in a gentle arc towards my other side.

'Get out!' shrieked the voice above my head. 'Get out, now!'

We both stood up awkwardly. The rose-covered door pushed against the fireman, forcing him hard against me, and the white door on my side thrust me painfully back. Clods of earth thumped around us and down on to Ivan's head which was now level with my ankles.

The earth trembled, and doors shifted again. 'Pull!' we screamed together, in unison with everyone who could see down into the hole.

A dozen pairs of arms, with a strength born of desperation, heaved on the rope. Ivan gave out a blood-curdling cry as, with an audible crack, his arm broke and came free. He rose two feet. His head was now level with my thigh and rammed hard into it.

'My leg!' he cried, weeping tears of pain, rage and impotence. 'It's caught.'

The earth moved again. The weight of the child on his pot crushed into my back.

'Pull!' we all screamed, and Ivan's leg gave way with a sickening crunching sound as he was yanked, like a cork from a bottle, out of his hole.

The fireman and I fought and scrabbled in fear as the sides of the hole finally fell in, pushing those two doors like the jaws of a vice inexorably together. Great lumps of earth fell down on top of them, and on us. As we climbed and fought our way up the cascading soil, dozens of hands, from ladders that we had not noticed across the top of the hole, reached down and pulled us up.

Ivan, who had fainted, had been laid on a stretcher. With shaking mud-covered hands, I tried to maintain a 'no touch' technique as I gave him a large injection of pain-killing morphine, and the two waiting ambulance men deftly applied splints to his arm and leg.

I sat exhausted on the wet earth as they loaded the stretcher into the ambulance and took him off to hospital.

I looked down into the hole. Where we had been, but moments before, was just a heap of earth. Had we not got out when we did, we would have been buried with Ivan three feet underneath it. I shuddered. Someone thrust a mug of hot sweet tea into my hands. Shaking like a leaf, I drank it.

The firemen around me began to gather up their gear in a calm and orderly manner, giving every appearance of satisfaction at another routine job well done. I sat and watched them, trying to work out which of them had been down the hole with me. I could not tell.

The officer came over, and thanked me for turning out. 'We damn' nearly didn't make it,' he said, automatically including me in the 'we' of his team.

'I'm damn' glad I don't have to do that every day,' I replied feelingly.

'Oh, you get used to it,' he said, and wandered off to see to his men.

Slowly I drove home. Wearily, I climbed the stairs to a hot bath, where I lay and soaked for over an hour. I had missed lunch, but food could wait until after my bath.

The boys wanted to resume digging for the blocked sewer pipe, but I told them firmly that I had been in enough holes for one day.

Still,' I said to Ruth, 'it gives us the perfect excuse to ask the council to keep using their tanker twice a week. We can't possibly have a new system until Ivan comes out of hospital, and it will probably be several months before he's fit to work again. We might have acquired some money by then.'

* * *

The following day, Monday, while paying my routine visit to the hospital, I went in to see Ivan. He was lying in a bed half-way down the ward. As I walked towards him, I

106

searched my memory for his proper name. It was on the tip of my tongue but would not come.

'Morning, there,' I said to him. One arm was encased in plaster from his finger-tips to his shoulder, and one leg from toes to thigh. His eyes were red and swollen, and a great bruised-looking weal ran diagonally across his face, disfiguring his nose.

He looked back at me expressionlessly. I could not tell whether this was due to absence of emotion or inflammation and swelling of his face. 'You look a damn' sight better than you did yesterday,' I said conversationally.

'Yes,' he agreed, 'should have known better, shouldn't I?'

'I'm sorry about that,' I said, pointing to his plasters, 'but we didn't really have much option, did we?'

'No,' he said, adding in a flat, croaky voice, 'Never thought that I'd ever thank anybody for breaking my arm in cold blood.' He paused. 'Nor for going on and doing my leg as well.'

'I'm sorry,' I said.

He got as near to a shrug of the shoulders as his plastered body would allow. 'Serves me right. But thanks, anyway.'

'How do you feel in yourself?'

'All right,' he replied, after a few moments. 'Bored to hell.'

'But you've only been here for a day,' I said.

'And that's a day too long,' he replied slowly and positively. 'Never was one for lying in bed. It's wasting time.'

'You're going to have to get used to it for a few days longer,' I told him. 'Can I get you anything to help you pass the time—some books or something?'

'No,' he said, without interest. 'No, thanks. Don't read books. Tried one once, when I was in the army, didn't get on with it.'

'Well, what do you do when you're not working?' I asked.

'Don't do anything else,' he replied, with just a touch of pride in his voice. 'I get bored when I'm not working.'

'You'll have to do something, other than just lie here,' I

107

said. 'No,' he disagreed, 'I'll just wait.'

As I left him, I did not know whether I envied him his simple life—a life apparently uncomplicated by emotions, feelings, anxieties and worries; a life of digging holes with brute strength, interrupted only by intervals of sleep, to regain that strength—or whether I felt sorry for him, sorry for all the beauty and imagination of this world, that he seemed to be missing.

He did not stay in the hospital long, and was sent out to mend his bones in his own bed. As he was not a patient of ours, I was not involved in his convalescence.

*   *   *

The passing weeks were recorded by the visits of the council tanker. They rang me once or twice, but seemed satisfied with my story of waiting for Ivan to recover, and kept us pumped out.

Financially, the tide was turning. Our overdraft was no longer going up. It seemed to have reached a high point, where it hovered for a long time, and had now receded a little, back to the figure that the friendly manager insisted was our absolute upper maximum.

Now that we had managed to regain that figure, I felt that, when Ivan came to give us his estimate, I could offer to pay him in instalments, but secretly I hoped that it would be several more months before we had to have the work done.

It was almost three months to the day when he walked up the drive, late one Sunday evening. He did not look as if he had ever been injured. His pace was his usual short-legged stride, and his arms were swinging freely. His face was unmarked.

'How are you, Ivan?' I asked, as I showed him into the kitchen. I still could not remember his real name.

'All right,' he said. I pointed to a chair at the table. 'Thanks,' he said as he sat down, 'it's still a bit stiff standing around.'

At that moment Ruth walked into the room and smiled a greeting at him. He took his cap off his bald head, put it down on the table and, very slightly embarrassed, said to her, 'Evening, Missis.'

The three of us sat at the table, for a moment in silence.

'Just come to let you know that I'll be starting on your job in the morning, Doc,' he said.

'But you haven't given us an estimate yet,' I exclaimed in surprise, 'and, to be honest, I don't know whether we'll be able to afford your bill all in one go.'

'There won't be any estimate,' he said flatly. 'Nor, for that matter, any bill, either.'

I stared at him in amazement. 'Don't be so damn' stupid,' I said at last. 'You said yourself that there's two weeks' work there, and God knows how much money in materials. You can't do that lot for nothing.'

He looked evenly back at me. 'You never sent me a bill for getting me out of that hole.'

'That's different,' I said. 'It's my job.'

'No different,' he replied. 'Putting sewers in is my job. I can charge what I like, and if I don't feel like charging . . .' He paused, and looked at me squarely. 'I don't feel like charging.'

'Don't be daft,' I tried again, 'this is your living.'

He cut across me. The look on his face, direct into mine, was disconcerting. 'What's the use of a living, Doc, if you haven't got a life to live it with?'

I stared at him in silence. I had nothing to say.

'Down that hole, Doc,' he said quietly, 'I died. Not . . .' trying hard to put his deep emotions into very inadequate words, 'not dead, as in a coffin dead, but me, here,' pointing with his finger into the middle of his chest. 'Me, I died in that hole.'

Neither Ruth nor I said anything.

'Never thought of dying before,' he continued in the same soft, musing voice, as if he was trying to express something incapable of being put into mere words, 'and it doesn't worry me now, not now that I've done it once.'

Ruth and I sat and waited.

'When my time comes for real, Doc,' and removing his gaze from my face, he looked down at the bare table. 'Just when it's all black and it's all over, the Good Lord will

109

reach down and catch hold of my hand.' He paused and opened and closed his fist, as if catching hold of that hand. 'He'll have a hand like yours, Doc. Warm, and soft and strong. And I'll hold that hand, knowing that it's never going to let me go, and I'm going to be all right.'

We all stared at the table.

'And then,' he said, 'will come the wonderful part. You know you're dying. You're alone, totally alone, and it's black and you're choking. And then'll come this glorious feeling of cold fresh air on your chest, that rises up till it's cold and fresh in your face, and as you breathe it in and breathe it in, you know that you're needed, and going up to Heaven.'

He stared at his hand, as it rubbed aimlessly up and down the table. A few moments went by.

'You'll know you're in Heaven, Doc, when He says in your ear, in that lovely soft voice, just like yours: "Ivan, we've got you now. You're OK".' He looked up at me. 'It won't matter that he can't recall that your name's Fred Shotton, he only knows you as Ivan the Terrible.'

I looked back at him. 'There'll be no charge, Doc,' he said.

Ruth rose quietly from her chair. 'Coffee or whisky?' she asked.

'Whisky,' I said.

She produced a fresh bottle and glasses, and silently, methodically and determinedly Ivan and I set about obliterating the memory of that hole.

*　*　*

Next morning, through red eyes and a thumping hangover, I was called by the children to the bedroom window.

A rusting, lumbering, ugly heap of mechanical digger creaked and groaned its way up to the top of the yard. It pushed out its legs and began to dig. Gracefully, the digging arm took a bite of earth and moved it to one side.

'It looks like a swan feeding,' Ruth said.

'Yes it does,' I agreed.

110

11

This particular member of the do-it-yourself duck breeding kit had a mind of her own. She was not inclined to co-operate.

She perched, high in her tree, quite out of reach, and looked down at me. Impotently I looked back, and swore; broody hens were not supposed to behave like this. More-over, those precious eggs she should have been sitting on were now getting cold, and I was already ten minutes late for my evening surgery.

With a derisive cackle, she jumped to a better and higher perch, from which she continued to peer balefully down at me.

The frustration within me exploded. Grabbing the only missile within reach, a half-brick, I vented my spleen. Fortunately for the hen, it hit the branch she was perched on. Had it connected, the force with which it was thrown would not only have killed that hen, but delivered her, plucked and oven-ready, at my feet. With a flurry of feathers, and squawking indignation, she disappeared over the horizon.

Perhaps we had been spoiled by the behaviour of the first of our motley collection of bantams to go broody. She had been a splendid little off-white creature, with soft hairy feathers that continued right down her legs and sprouted out between her toes. She was placid, confiding and maternal, and fully convinced in her little mind that her only function in life was to sit on eggs and keep them warm.

She had gone broody within a very short time after arriving at her new home, sitting regally and serene in one of the two nesting boxes that we had put in the pen, while the other hens had climbed in beside her to deposit ever more eggs for her attention. Each egg she had pulled positively underneath her with her beak, so that every evening, when we went to feed, she was sitting on a veritable mountain of them.

With the aid of a picture in a magazine, *The Smallholder and Beekeeper*, 'published weekly'—this particular copy being the issue for 7th March, 1923—Andrew and his friend Alex set about making a sitting box. The magazine had been provided by Alex's grandfather who, according to Alex, was the ultimate fount of knowledge on anything to do with broody hens. Unfortunately for our further education, Alex's grandfather lived in an old folk's home up Swaffham way, and his memory was not what it had been. The only reason the magazine had been kept at all was that Grandfather had written to the editor, pointing out that his theories on American Foul Brood were erroneous, and the letter had been published. The fact that Foul Brood is a disease of bees, and that Grandfather had never kept a hen in his life, was deemed by all parties to be singularly irrelevant.

But the magazine did contain an article on the manufacture and siting of sitting boxes for broody hens, and tips for controlling the humidity within them. It could be reduced to a single sentence: any old box would do, with a shovelful of moist earth in it covered by a handful of straw.

The boys were deputed to make such a box and, with much pomp and ceremony, Henrietta, as she had now become, was duly transferred, together with her pile of eggs. In the fullness of time—nineteen days, to be exact—she hatched every one.

It seemed so easy; we could hardly wait until the duck breeding season started. Armed with rows and rows of sitting Henriettas, we would hatch every egg they laid.

It did not work out like that at all. Most of those hens were not Henriettas, they were Harridans, with cruel eyes and vicious beaks, mean and evil-tempered, and distinctly non co-operative as far as duck egg hatching was concerned. The one at which I had just hurled the half-brick was typical of the species: long-legged, long-tailed, and as black in her character as her straggly feathers; as far as I was concerned, she could stay where she had landed, two fields away, and the sooner a fox ate her the better.

112

In the meantime, however, I had to find some other place to keep those eggs warm, and calm myself down to deal with another packed and now exceedingly late surgery. The airing cupboard in the kitchen was the obvious place to put the eggs; indeed, it had been used before in such dire circumstances, as an emergency sanctuary. Unfortunately, it was temporarily out of action, a casualty of the do-it-yourself mania for home improvements, aided and abetted by a primary school teacher who fancied himself as an amateur plumber.

Desperately, I searched both the house and my mind for somewhere else, warm and safe, where I could put those eggs.

Memories surfaced on reading in a book somewhere, that South African ostrich farmers paid their native girls to hatch these enormous eggs tucked under their commodious bosoms. Places adequate for ostrich eggs would, I reasoned, surely hold a few duck eggs in comfort, at least overnight, while we waited for that black-hearted monster to return, or for another hen to go broody.

Fortunately for the sanctity of our marriage, Ruth had gone into town shopping, with all the children, to buy them all yet more pairs of new shoes. They each had such differing widths of feet and such total disregard for where they put them, that handing any outgrown shoes down the family could not happen. I knew from bitter experience that she would be shopping until closing time, and something deep inside me said that, on her return, it would be better not to make such a proposal seriously.

But somehow I had to keep those eggs warm. With a bit of luck, the primary school plumber would help me get the airing cupboard back in working order during the evening, and the warmth of a female cleavage would be needed for only a few hours.

There was no other hen sitting in the shed, that I could use, nowhere suitable or warm enough inside the house; so I did the only thing that came to mind, that was compatible with going off to do the evening surgery: I put those precious eggs inside my own shirt and gingerly drove off to work. Not being anatomically equipped to keep a clutch

113

of eggs stable as well as warm, they rolled about something alarming, but it would have to do.

Our receptionist was very new and very efficient. We had grave difficulty keeping receptionists. Although neither Mac nor I had anything to do with it physcially, there seemed to be something about working for us that enhanced their fertility. Even quite respectable matrons soon developed that broody look and, grinning coyly, gave us notice. The succession became embarrassing, and a source of great amusement to our medical colleagues.

The present one had been chosen not for her good looks, but because she had been married for ten childless years, and her husband was in the navy.

I walked in vey carefully, with the eggs in my shirt, bag in one hand and folders of notes tucked under the other arm. She looked up at me from behind her desk, ostentatiously glanced at her watch and reached out for the folder of notes. With all those eggs hovering delicately around my umbilicus, I dared not bend to put my case on the floor. I edged closer so that she could reach the notes under my arm.

'You're late again, Doctor,' she remarked. 'Your patients may have become used to it, but I have not.'

I surveyed her as she sat there, plump, comfortable and well-endowed, with plenty of room for all those eggs in my shirt, but with something of the same air about her as that black hen.

'I do not intend to be late tonight,' she informed me.

'Sorry,' I said meekly. Tonight was certainly not the night to ask her to keep my eggs warm in her bra.

I do not know whether any of the patients that night found my behaviour a trifle odd, but it did require the skill of a tightrope artist to rise from my chair without bending in the middle, and to lean forward over the couch, using only my ankles and knees. Several times, between patients, I had to rearrange those eggs, bringing the cooler ones in from the outside to be warmed in the middle. I hoped that no one was aware of the increasingly pungent aroma of henhouse that seemed to become ever stronger as the evening wore on.

114

Eventually I finished that surgery, not too late by my standards but late enough to get a very frosty look from that receptionist, waiting to file the last of the notes away. I did not tell her about the eggs in my shirt.

Driving home, I realised why she reminded me so much of that black-hearted hen. She, too, had gone unwillingly broody and had all the outward signs of early pregnancy. Her basic hormones were dragging her reluctant intellect behind them. Something must have gone wrong the last time her naval husband was around. No doubt, within a few weeks, she would admit it and give us notice. I would not really be sorry to see her go.

Back home, the crisis was over. That much-maligned hen had returned to her nest and was sitting, as good as gold. With great relief, I handed the eggs over to Ruth who placed them gently back under the hen, without any fuss whatsoever.

'I think,' she said tactfully over supper, 'that you had better let me handle the broodies, while you restore the hot water system.'

'Yes, dear,' I said.

* * *

While we were still eating, Neville, the schoolmaster, arrived. With his usual enthusiasm he bounced into the room, festooned with his plumbing tools and miles of assorted sizes of second-hand water pipes. He had enjoyed a very successful day touring the scrap heaps of every builder in town.

Although now in his early thirties, he had an air of Peter Pan about him, enhanced by his large clear glasses forever falling forward down his nose, and his rapidly receding blond hair. He had the enthusiasm of a small boy, which was exceedingly contagious, whether he was demonstrating to his class his home-made model of how the tide came in, or, in this case, demonstrating to his medical adviser, in a very practical manner, how to warm up a cold bathroom.

Our bathroom had been installed, as an afterthought, some time in the 1890s, on the coldest, north-east corner of

115

the house. An old boiler, in an outhouse in the garden, coughed and wheezed black soot into the prevailing wind as it tried to warm the house. There was no central heating upstairs, and hot water appeared from a very devious and complicated system of pipes leading to and from the airing cupboard in the kitchen.

Neville was an instant expert. He carried the natural air of knowing a great deal more about everything than any of the children in his class, into the greater world outside his school. What he did not know, he could soon find out from one of the many do-it-yourself manuals or encyclopaedias lining his bookshelves, or from the informative reporting in the weightier Sunday newspapers. Anything, from making an atomic bomb to extending an ancient and defunct central heating system, was within his grasp. All he needed was the instruction book, the time and the materials.

He had informed me, very proudly, some months before, that he had now completed the installation of his own central heating system, and how pleased he was with the result. Misguidedly, I had told him of the rigours of taking a bath in the arctic conditions of our newly acquired bathroom.

He had stared at me in total amazement, across the surgery desk.

'But that's easy to sort out,' he stated confidently. 'All you need is to fix a spur off the main pipes and run it up to your bathroom.'

'And a radiator, and all the fittings, and all the holes in the walls,' I added dubiously. I had grave doubts of the wisdom of disturbing all those ancient lime-encrusted pipes, particularly when done by enthusiastic amateurs. 'Besides which, it's far too cold at the moment to turn the system off. It's a summer job.'

'Leave it with me,' he replied. 'I've got a lot of pipes left over from my system. I'll get the radiator and the fittings, hire one of those big wall drills, and as soon as the weather warms up, we'll do it.'

That had been some months ago. I had forgotten all about the conversation, but Neville had not. He had

116

arrived unexpectedly one evening, raring to go. Everything, but everything, had to stop. No matter what it was, it had to take second place to fitting a radiator in the bathroom.

I had to agree with him, as he pointed out just how simple and straightforward it was. Turn off the water, drain the system, cut out sections of pipe here and here, insert the take-off junctions, and screw in the new pipes to the bathroom.

First, turn off the water. It took us most of the first evening to find the stop tap, and most of the second hammering and oiling it, to get it to turn. Eventually we managed to stop the flow of water into the pipes sufficiently to turn our attentions to the tap that drained the system, and run it off. That was nearly as bad, but finally Neville deemed it empty enough to begin cutting out his sections of pipe. Underneath multiple layers of paint and rust, they were not the soft copper he was expecting, but hard, thick, black steel, as hard and as black as the hearts of that hen and our new receptionist combined. It was not until he had cut half-through one of them that he realised his junctions would not fit. They were all brass and copper, and he needed the old-fashioned cast-iron sort.

Completely undeterred, he left us waterless, with a promise to return the next night with junctions of the right type, and had actually cut out the sections of pipe before he discovered that his new ones were no better than his old. They had to be screwed on, and he had not got a tool to put the right threads on the old pipes.

Tonight, he had returned with what he confidently expected to be the right equipment, all of it scrounged from assorted rubbish dumps.

He was dispatched to fit his junctions, while we finished eating. The job went deceptively smoothly. By the time that I joined him, they were in, with ends of string and red lead hanging out all over the place, while he heaved and braced the spanners on the joints.

'That's the difficult part done,' he grinned, boyish and triumphant. 'Now for the easy bit.'

He ran an extension cable from the plug in the hall,

mounted a chair and thrust his massive hired electric masonry drill into the ceiling. It sank effortlessly out of sight into the plaster, there was an explosive flash and a bang, and all the lights went out. The drill stopped, too, leaving Neville hanging from it and wobbling precariously on his chair. A large chunk of ceiling slowly detached itself from the rest, and ceiling, drill, Neville and chair unceremoniously became a tangled mass on the floor.

He sat up and grinned at me through the gloom and the dust. 'Good job this drill's double-insulated. Never felt a thing.'

I looked up at the ceiling. Even in this poor light, I could see that he had cut the main cable neatly in half.

Somehow, from somewhere, we found a junction box, connected the severed wires to it and replaced the blown main fuse. I was quite prepared to call that enough for one night, but not Neville. His boy-scout mentality insisted that we finish the job we had set out to do. Mounting his chair once more, and with the aid of the newly restored light, he thrust his drill up and through the bathroom floor.

A motley assortment of short lengths of pipe were soon joined together and poked up through the holes. We surveyed their ends upstairs in the bathroom. Ruth regarded them quizzically. Very unwisely she spoke her thoughts.

'Now you've made so much mess,' she began tentatively, 'wouldn't it be better if you moved the radiator over here, by the window?'

'No,' I said emphatically.

'What a good idea,' enthused my far-from-favourite boy scout. 'If we pull up those floor-boards, I can run the pipes underneath them and make a really neat job of it.'

I was outvoted two to one; had I known what was to follow, I would not have allowed myself to be so easily over-ruled. I did, however, insist that, at least for tonight, those pipe ends be capped with the old steel radiator Neville had scrounged, so that the water could be reconnected to the boiler and I could have a bath. I stank of henhouse, was sweaty and dusty, and had no desire to repeat the egg-warming manoeuvre again, for want of an airing

118

cupboard.

After the radiator had been connected, we tentatively turned the water back on and lit the boiler. That hot bath was sheer bliss; I even mellowed a little in my attitude to that black hen. If she misbehaved, I had the warm airing cupboard back in reserve.

At least, I thought I had. Neville had other ideas. He intended to make a proper job of heating our bathroom, and arrived the next night with yet more second-hand plumbing, and his second wind in enthusiasm.

Before I could stop him, he was upstairs and ripping up the bathroom floor-boards.

'Good job the joists run this way,' he grinned up at me, as I opened my mouth to speak. 'Won't have to take up all the boards to get the pipes through.'

Pushing his spectacles back up his nose again, he ambled over to the far wall, knelt down and began probing the cracks with a massive screwdriver. 'Gottcha,' he said, as he levered on it, and protesting nails, comfortably rusted into the old wood for at least the last half-century, squealed as they were forcibly withdrawn.

One end of the plank came up easily, the other remained firmly fixed, where the entire weight of the bath rested on it. Neville pushed back his spectacles and reached for the saw.

'You're not going to cut it,' I said aghast.

'Sure,' he grinned at me. 'How else do I get it out of the way?'

At that moment the telephone rang and I left him, to answer it. Walking into the bedroom, I picked up the instrument. My mind was distracted from the voice by the sounds of vigorous sawing. With visions of our bath lurching to a three-legged position at an angle to the floor, I tried to concentrate on old Fred Scoggins and his problem.

*   *   *

Fred was a trial both to himself and to me. Although now well into his seventies, he still worked an eighteen-hour day in his little corner shop. When he had first joined the

119

business as a lad of fourteen, his father had proudly painted 'Scoggins and Son' over the shop window, and there it had remained ever since. It was somewhat faded and peeling now, but still visible. Old Father Scoggins had lived and worked to a ripe old age, and during all this time Fred had never advanced from his position as errand boy. He was well into his fifties by the time his father died and left him the shop, and somehow had never got round to marrying. He was a fussy little bachelor, the original 'old maid'. Over the years, trade had slowly drifted down, so that he could not afford either to employ staff or to retire. I had suggested to him many times that if he sold the shop, he could buy a small bungalow and live in comfort. All my suggestions had been gently but firmly rejected.

'Just before he died, my father asked me to make no change,' he reminded me.

For some months now he had been in mild heart failure, a diagnosis made only too easy from his wheezy chest, swollen ankles and irregular pulse. He was also acutely embarrassed by his old man's complaint of the need to pass his water every hour or so.

Whenever he needed medical attention, he always waited until evening to contact me, after he had shut his shop for the day.

He had summoned me a few nights previously.

'I know how busy we both are during the day, Doctor,' he had said diffidently into the 'phone, 'so I thought I'd leave asking you to come and see me till we had both finished, and had got time to deal with my problem properly.'

I had examined him thoroughly, the more intimate parts of which had caused him almost to die of shame.

He had gazed at me reproachfully, after I had assessed the size of his prostate and as he was replacing his trousers. 'That must surely be the ultimate indignity,' he said sadly.

I had warned him that the pills I was about to give him, to clear the congestion from his chest, would cause him to pass considerably more water than usual; so much so, that there was a high probability he would develop a complete retention of his water and need an operation to relieve it.

'Ooh, no, Doctor,' he said disbelievingly, 'I have no intention of going into hospital at my age. I'm too old for things like that now. Father never had any faith in hospitals, he told me repeatedly never to set foot in one.'

I had left him with his prescription, and the feeling that he would not take any of the pills for fear that his father would have disapproved.

Now he was telling me, over the 'phone, in competition with the sounds of the destruction of my bathroom, that he, too, had the predicted plumbing problems. He had cashed the prescription, but it had taken him three days to pluck up courage to take a pill. The first dose had eased his shortness of breath considerably for several hours, but when it had recurred, with courage in both hands and making apologies to his father, he had taken a double dose of everything. The expected result had happened: the sudden shifting of fluid from his lungs to his bladder had overfilled it, and he was now in considerable and increasing discomfort, quite unable to pass his water at all.

Silently cursing him, I told him to hang on, and I would come as soon as I could. Putting down the 'phone, I walked apprehensively back to the bathroom, from which emanated an ominous silence. Neville was surveying the wreckage.

'Bit of a problem with the plumbing, Doc,' he muttered, as he peered into what had once been our bathroom floor. From his kneeling position, he looked at me over his shoulder and pushed the spectacles back up his nose. 'I think those pipes are blocked.'

'Don't tell me.' I stopped his gesticulating explanation. 'I've got a panic call. Some old boy's got *his* plumbing blocked, and I've got to get that sorted out. Carry on, and I'll be back as soon as I can.'

I drove to Old Fred's corner shop. He was in the back room, pacing slowly up and down, with his legs wide apart and an expression of acute misery on his face.

Reluctantly, at my request, he went upstairs, undressed, and lay on his bed. The pain of his unrelieved bladder was as nothing compared to the shame of expos-

121

ing himself to another person. Nobody, but nobody, had gazed on that part of his anatomy since his mother had last changed his nappies, let alone passed a large rubber catheter up it.

Eventually the job was done, but although the pain had been relieved, his whole demeanour indicated strongly that his person had been defiled and that he would never be the same again.

I left him, with the catheter still in place and with full instructions how to remove the spigot to empty his bladder himself, and went back to my own plumbing problems.

By now, Neville had moved the radiator and was hammering the floor-boards back into place. I did not enquire which pipes had been blocked.

The water was turned back on, the boiler re-lit, and all appeared to be well. I heaved sighs of relief and thought of a lovely hot bath.

'What you really need in here now,' Neville said to Ruth as we surveyed the distinctly irregular levels of the hammered-back floor-boards, 'are some nice cork tiles.' He went down on his knees and, enthusiatically pushing his spectacles back up his nose, eyed the boards.

'If we nail plywood over the whole floor first, it'll be a lovely finish.'

I groaned, but I was outvoted.

'Can't come tomorrow.' He paused, just a trifle bashful. 'I've got to go out.'

'You're not courting,' I grinned at him. Neville was another confirmed bachelor. He had told me many times that he was waiting for the right girl to come along, but never seemed to make any effort to look for her.

Blushing, he poked awkwardly at his glasses with an embarrassed finger. I stared at him in amazement.

'What's her name? Do we know her?'

'Er, yes, er no.' He looked more like a great big overgrown schoolboy than ever. 'When I get the plywood, I'll get some ceiling boards for downstairs at the same time.'

I did not press him. The last thing I had expected was an admission that he was going courting; besides, it would be nice to have a few evenings free from his enthusiastic alterations of our house.

He gathered up his tools. 'I'll see you in a few days,' he said as he went out of the door.

The few days turned out to be over a week. The bathroom was nice and warm, the hole in the cloakroom ceiling did not bother me overmuch, that black hen was impeccably behaved, and several more hens went broody. Even our receptionist's frosty manner melted a little. Mac and I discussed it. We were both agreed that she gave out all the familiar outward signs of early pregnancy, but he was adamant that the sailor husband had not been home for over a year. Deciding that it was none of our business, we agreed to do and say nothing until she gave us notice.

*   *   *

Old Fred crept into the surgery one morning and announced that he had shut his shop and was ready for his operation. Over the 'phone, I explained his predicament to the surgeon who agreed to admit him straight away.

'Make a new man of you,' I said, trying to cheer him up.

Miserably, he shook his head. 'Don't know what Father would say.' Those tired old eyes appealed to me. 'I feel I've broken faith with him, but I haven't any choice, have I?'

'No,' I agreed, as he shuffled out dejectedly.

Neville exploded into the kitchen that evening, as usual while we were eating, half-carrying, half-dragging sheets of plywood. He looked as if he was bursting to say something, but changed his mind and went outside again for more.

I helped him carry it all up the stairs, cut it to shape round the various bathroom fittings, and nail it to the floor. It was well into the night before we had finished. His usual exuberance was strangely muted, less of a little boy on a great adventure, more a man in a hurry to get done. Our conversation was confined purely to the technicalities of fitting the wood, but several times I felt that he was on the point of telling me a great secret; however, he did not.

The next evening, we laid the cork tiles, meticulously

123

according to the instruction book. Neville enthused, bounced and corrected, but the subtle change was still there. We admired the finished work.

'Er,' said Neville, pushing his spectacles back up his nose once more, but he never finished the sentence. The moment passed, and the conversation turned to the hole in the ceiling below. We agreed that the only way we could mend it was to rip out the whole of the old plasterboard and replace it with a new piece.

This he did, the following night. I was unable to help him; I was late coming in, and the telephone rang non-stop. When I did finally finish, Neville had gone home. He had spent the entire evening pulling down the old ceiling and trying to put back all the electrical fittings that had fallen out.

It took us two more whole evenings to replace that ceiling and plaster it in, a process not helped by cutting the holes for the ceiling switches in the wrong places. Rather more force than was good for it was applied to the already taut wiring, to make it reach our holes, but eventually the job was done and we stood admiring our handiwork.

'Can you manage the painting yourself?' asked Neville hopefully. 'I, er, shall be rather busy for the next few weeks.'

'You're not still courting, are you?' I teased him.

He pushed those spectacles firmly back up his nose. 'Yes,' he said, almost defiantly. 'We're getting married next week.'

We stared at him in amazement. 'That's rushing things a bit, even for you, isn't it?' I said eventually.

'Well, yes,' he admitted slowly. Then all of a sudden, almost bouncing back to his usual self, 'We've sort of got to, if you see what I mean, and you're going to need a new receptionist.'

He grinned at me, and the glasses went back up his nose again. 'So she's the lucky lady,' I said. 'But hang on a minute, isn't she married already, to some chap in the navy?'

'Was,' he corrected. 'They were divorced over a year ago. She didn't like talking about it, so never told any-

124

body.'

He bounced out of our house, and was gone.

It was much later that evening that we discovered none of the lights worked in the bathroom. Neville's energetic pulling, to get the wires to fit his holes, had pulled them out of the junction box. I knew exactly where it was; the problem was, should I rip out the floor or the ceiling to get at it?

It took me two weeks to decide to rip up the floor and fix it. It was finally done on the day that Neville and our ex-receptionist got married, the day Old Fred came out of hospital, and the day on which that black-hearted hen hatched out her duck eggs and became a model mother.

12

'This is ridiculous,' I said. 'We've got to automate this time-consuming process somehow.'

'I'd like to see you try,' Ruth replied indignantly, as she lifted off another hen. 'How can you automate a shed full of broody hens?'

'I don't know,' I replied, 'but I'm going to have a damn' good try.' The hens sat on the floor and I went off to think about it—or rather, I went off to work and hoped that my subconscious would think about it, while the rest of my brain was busy with everything else. I had lots of problems on my mind at that moment.

For a start, our friendly bank manager had gone down with jaundice and was taking a long time to get over it. He would make a full recovery in time, and apart from having to give up his favourite alcoholic drink for six months, would be none the worse eventually. The problem was his deputy. He was not nearly so friendly, and was taking an unhealthy interest in our overdraft. I had explained to him that although, like his jaundiced manager, our bank account was sick, the illness was not terminal. Given the same treatment—sufficient time, plenty of good food and exercise—it would recover eventually. He disagreed. His views were more those of the surgeon: that bad debt was corrupting and should be removed at once. We were still arguing over the treatment and there had been another letter from him that morning.

Secondly, I had belly aches all over town that I was sitting on, or in more medical terms, keeping under observation. There seemed to be a positive epidemic of them at the moment. A straightforward appendicitis, where the signs and symptoms are clear-cut, is not a cause for worry; it is a simple job of work. Similarly, where the pain is caused by colic, of the eating-too-many-green-apples variety, there is no cause for worry; it will get better on its own, and one of Grandmother's homely remedies will ease the misery until it passes. The problem ones were those where the diagnosis was not instantly obvious, and I had to let a little time pass by and see what developed.

There had been one yesterday, which had presented as a painful but simple overdue period in a young girl of fifteen. Despite her strenuous denial of possible pregnancy, and the indignation that such questioning had provoked from her mother, the alarm bells had rung in my brain. Against my instinctive better judgement, I had sat on her and awaited events. Her ectopic pregnancy had ruptured late that afternoon, with almost fatal results.

I was sitting on several other such time bombs, most of which were harmless, but any one of which could explode under me at any moment. If only I knew which, there would be no cause for worry, as I could defuse them by putting them into hospital. It was a great pity that I could not hospitalise the lot, but that would only have the effect of blocking every bed in the place and bringing the whole system to a standstill.

The third and most important worry was that my good wife was spending six hours of every day seeing to her broody hens, and changing the food and water pots of all those little ducks. The household was beginning to suffer, with such symptoms as no clean clothes for the children, and no dinner for me. But, as I had agreed, the ducks came first. We needed the money that they represented.

To employ someone to do it was the obvious answer, but they would need paying. A very simple calculation showed that the wages required would come to more than the ducks would yield, and there was also the unresolved problem of the unsympathetic deputy bank manager.

The only practical solution was to automate the hatching and rearing and cut out all the work. But how? That was the problem. I would let my subconscious work on it, while I grappled with all those belly aches and composed a suitable reply to the latest demands from the bank.

*   *   *

'Let me make a suggestion,' said the good Leslie Warner, the first patient of the day, across the surgery desk.

He was one of the time bombs I had been sitting on. His pain was gall bladder colic, but the special X-ray last week had shown that he had only a single gall stone. As his pain had settled, we both hoped that he had passed it himself, and today's X-ray showed that it had definitely gone. He would not need an operation to remove it, and we were both much relieved.

He always prefaced every proposed action with the words, 'Let me make a suggestion', whether the action proposed was to arrange an X-ray, or to transport some surplus bantam cockerels to market.

He had appeared in the yard one day, soon after we had acquired the bantams, driving his battered old car with the inevitable old trailer hooked behind it.

'I hear that you have some unwanted bantam cockerels,' he said. How he came by the information I never did discover; the village grapevine must have been super-efficient. 'Let me make a suggestion,' he said. 'I have a friend who has asked me to find him some bantam cockerels. I will take the lot, he can choose the ones he wants, and I'll take the rest to market.'

That had been the first of many such transactions. He had returned from the market with a few pence for us and, thereafter, whenever we wanted anything, Leslie was always the first person that we asked.

And now, with the shadow of an impending gall bladder operation removed, the relief on his weatherbeaten old face was gratifying; I had done the correct thing by sitting on him. He knew all about the vast amount of work that the ducks involved, and how I was trying to make it more manageable. 'Let me make a suggestion,' he repeated. 'I have a friend who used to breed turkeys. He's not been well for a year or two, and I know that he used to have several incubators. I'm sure if we went to see him, he would let you have one.'

'That sounds like a good idea,' I replied, 'but we shall still need the broody hens for rearing the ducks. What takes the time is constantly refilling the food and water pots, and moving the runs on to fresh grass.'

'I know,' he said. 'I have watched it all coming along.'

* * *

It had been great fun at first, watching all the courting antics of the various ducks, and predicting which duck would be the first to lay. Just before they come into lay, the tail ends of the ducks enlarge, so that they become very heavy and bulbous between their legs. If a duck in that condition did not come up at feeding time, it was a fair bet that it had a nest somewhere.

The bantams, too, had been laying like mad. We had eggs everywhere, and as soon as any bantam had gone broody and wanted to sit on eggs, we had let it; so we now had hens and chicks everywhere.

When the first clutches of duck eggs began to appear, there was not a single broody hen spare. Every evening I went into the hen run and looked into the nesting boxes for a sitting hen. If a hen is sitting in the box by day, it is probably just laying an egg, but if it is still sitting there at night, it has either gone broody, or else it may be just too lazy to perch and is merely having a comfortable sleep.

We discovered very early on how to tell which was which, by putting a hand underneath the hen. If it flew off squawking, it was no good, but if it sat and tolerated the hand, there was promise. If the hand was then turned palm upwards, and the fingers gently pushed into the breast of the bird, a genuine broody would ruffle its feathers, emit the characteristic broody noise, and try to settle the finger ends into a more comfortable position to sit on.

Night after night I had gone into the shed, but there were nothing but false alarms and temporarily raised hopes. Even if I found a broody, it would have to sit undisturbed for several days, as moving it to a sitting box prematurely could put it off and send it back to laying more eggs before it thought of going broody again.

I knew that we definitely had several clutches of eggs down on the island, ready to be picked up and put under a hen. There was one in particular, that of the little Carolina

129

Wood Duck which had made a nest in one of the boxes that we had put down there. From the entrance hole in the box a trail of silvery white down poured in all directions, with no intention of disguising the nest site from the eyes of ever-waiting predators. The male, a glorious study in purple and golden brown, erected his green shining crest at us whenever we went too near.

We knew the nest was vulnerable, but we had no broody hen.

One evening the inevitable happened. The light of the summer day had almost gone when John came downstairs.

'Dad,' he said, 'I think there are some people running about the island.'

I rushed to the window but could see nothing, so went out to look, and to my horrow saw a gang of youths running away to the gate behind the island. As I raced after them, the straggler came over the bridge, well behind the others, and I just managed to catch him with a rugby tackle as he raced for his bike. We both fell hard onto the earth, with him underneath.

He had my entire clutch of Carolina Wood Duck eggs in his shirt. Every one of the half-developed eggs was smashed. None too gently, I hauled him to his feet by the scruff of his neck and, with the mess of blood and yolk dripping from his waistband, marched him up to the house and 'phoned for Peter, our local policeman.

He walked him the five miles to the police station where his parents were summoned. They came out to apologise, and like a fool I did not press charges, even though the raid had cost us several hundred pounds in damage.

When Leslie called a few days later, in the hope of some surplus bantam eggs, I told him all about it.

'If I may make a suggestion,' he said, 'my old dad used to be a gamekeeper, and when he had problems like this, he used to leave a whole lot of old and rotten eggs about, in dummy nests, and hope that they'd be content with them and not find the real ones.'

Like most of his suggestions, it was a good one, and that is what we did, as well as removing most of the eggs from the nests as we found them, replacing them with either

130

mallard, bantam or pigeon eggs, depending on their size.

About two weeks later, again as it was just getting dark, there was a tap on my study window. My study was on the far side of the house from the island, and also from the back door. It was Leslie.

'I was just passing, Doc,' he said, 'and saw a whole lot of bikes hidden in the hedge just up the road. I have taken the precaution of putting them all in my trailer, and it would seem that their owners are all down on your island.'

'Thanks,' I said. 'I'll go and catch the little sods,' and I started to run out of the room and down to the island.

'If I may make a suggestion,' and I stopped and went back to the window. 'I have their bicycles, and I've parked my car round the corner. They don't know I've got them. Telephone for the police force, then when you go out to them, we shall be waiting where they left their bikes.'

I did exactly as he said, and when I saw the police car go past, I set off for the island. As soon as I appeared at the back door, the gang left the island in a hurry and raced off to their bikes, with me in hot pursuit. They must have had nearly a hundred yards' start, and there were no stragglers to catch.

When I caught them up, the two policemen and Leslie had them all lined up on the roadside. The smell of rotten eggs rose in the still evening. Leslie was doing a thorough search by slapping every pocket, to ensure that it contained no eggs and, if it felt suspicious, giving it a thorough going over.

The last one in the line frantically dug in his pockets, presenting the eggs to Leslie who, after inspecting them to make sure that they were suitable, took off the boy's cap, filled it with the eggs and replaced it firmly on his head, giving it a smart pat as he did so.

'There, boy,' he said, 'it always pays to own up.'

The smell was overpowering. They must have had over a hundred rotten eggs between them, and Leslie was not satisfied until he had dealt with every one. 'Take them away,' he said to the policemen. 'This time we are preferring charges, aren't we, Doc?'

'Go on, start walking,' said Peter, pointing up the road

131

to the town.

'What about my bike?' whined one of them.

'What about it?' Leslie replied. 'You stole all our valuable eggs and smashed them. The bikes have been confiscated and will be sold, to help pay for the damage you've done. Go on, get walking.'

We watched them head off up the road, a miserable, stinking rabble. Like a sheepdog, the police car followed behind, herding them on.

'Thank you,' I said to Leslie. 'Without you, they would have just run away and come back tomorrow. I don't think that they'll be back after that.'

'May I make a suggestion? Lock their bikes in a shed, and make them come back one at a time to collect them and apologise personally. When they come, give each boy a guided tour, show him every duck, and explain what you're doing. Tell him how much each duck cost. If you do that, you won't get any further trouble, the word will spread.'

Leslie's suggestions were, as far as I was concerned, royal commands. I saw every boy, and each one meant it when he apologised. We had no further trouble that year.

*   *   *

The advice about the incubators must also be taken seriously. I looked back at him across the surgery desk.

'Tell me about these incubators,' I said.

'Let me make a suggestion. Wednesday is your day off. I'll take you over to see them.'

I had got other plans, but it was a royal command.

We drove over in his battered old car, with the trailer oscillating behind. His friend lived up a narrow, bumpy little track, but he did not change speed, and the trailer leaped up and down as well as sideways. I felt sorry for any poor chicken he took anywhere in it; it would arrive quite seasick. Eventually we arrived at the farmyard.

At first, I thought the place was unoccupied, it looked totally derelict—grass a foot high grew in the drive, and the door to the barn had fallen off years ago, with stinging nettles and thistles growing round and through it. The plaster as well as the paint was peeling off the walls of the house, and there was only a trace of a path through the shoulder-high weeds to the front door.

Leslie surveyed it with dismay. 'Poor old sod. This used to be one of the neatest turkey breeding units in the country. He hasn't got long, poor old sod.'

He knocked on the door, called out a cheery greeting and walked straight in. I followed quietly behind. The old man sat in his chair by the electric fire. His clothes were dirty and unkempt, and a pile of untouched sandwiches and an unopened bottle of beer sat on the table. The sandwiches had obviously been there some time; they were beginning to curl at the edges. Sightlessly he stared at us, his old eyes milky-white with cataracts. His voice was not strong, as he called out,

'Who's that, then? Speak up, so I'll know who you are.'

Leslie identified himself and grasped the old man's hand. They remained like that for several moments.

'It's good to see you, boy,' he said, and did not release his hold. 'You've come to see me before I die.' He was completely unaware of my presence, and I felt that I was intruding.

They talked of old times, and a good half-hour had gone by before the old man said to him, 'Now tell me what you've come for. You never come unless you want something. What is it this time?'

Leslie smiled and chided the old man. 'Let me make a suggestion. I have a young man breeding ornamental ducks, and he needs an incubator. Yours out in that shed are the best. If you're not using them this season, can he borrow one to tide him over?'

'He can have the lot,' the old man replied. 'You know I'll never use them again. Only . . .' he paused, and as he spoke, he seemed to sag and lose a little of his bearing, 'tell him to look after them. They've been good to me, and if he treats them well, they'll be good to him.'

'Thanks,' said Leslie, rising from his chair. 'I'll go and load them into my trailer, and I'll pop back before I go.'

I was glad he had not mentioned my presence and

tiptoed out behind him.

We crossed the yard to the incubator shed, behind the main barn. The roof of the building had caved in over half its length some time previously, and there was no sign of any door. We walked into the wreckage. The incubators were the old-fashioned wooden table type, standing on legs and heated by a paraffin flame. There had originally been more than a dozen in the shed, but those exposed to the elements were a sorry sight.

With broken legs, they lurched at all angles, and from every joint in the woodwork grass and other plants grew in profusion. One stood upright. I tried to open the front of it and, as I pulled, the legs gave way and it crashed to the floor, spilling dirt and rotten wood as it did so. There were only three that had stayed in the dry, and in these the woodworms were having a field day. Their entire structure was completely riddled with them. One fell to pieces as we tried to open it, but there seemed sufficient left of the other two to warrant loading them into the trailer. They were put in gingerly, upside down, for the legs would never stand the journey. For luck we added a few extra paraffin containers, wicks and chimneys, in case the ones on the relatively intact machines were too full of rust to use.

After it had all been loaded up, Leslie took me into the old rearing shed. Hanging from the roof were hundreds of infra-red heating bulbs, all connected by yards and yards of electrical wiring, and as many small automatic drinkers, joined together by small-bore plastic tubing.

'If I may make a suggestion,' he said, 'my good friend has no further use for them. Take some and use them to rear your ducks, instead of the hens.' Without further ado, he disconnected a couple of dozen of each and put them with the rest in the trailer.

I felt rather like a vulture eating carrion.

Walking back to the house to say goodbye to the old man, I said to Leslie, 'I must pay for them. Please don't haggle with him over the price. Give him whatever he asks for,' and he nodded his agreement.

Leslie told him what we had taken, but did not tell him

134

of the state of dereliction. 'How much do we owe you?' he asked.

'My old friend,' came the reply, 'we have known each other a long time. We both know money is no good to me, I can't take it with me. Tell your young man that if he doesn't take care of them, I will come and haunt him. I've not got long and, to be honest, going will be a relief. Tell him he can have them with my compliments. It's comforting to know that someone else will make use of them.'

I felt less like a carrion eater and was glad that he did not know of my presence. It was better between just the two old friends, and Leslie would thank him on my behalf, far better than I could personally.

'May I make a suggestion?' he said after he had done so. 'You're here all alone, with no one to look after you. Why don't you move to somewhere where you can be waited on and looked after?'

'No,' he said. 'We've been through all that before. I've had my life here, and it's my home. Just leave me be and let me go, among my memories, in peace and with dignity.'

We left him, alone with his dignity, his unopened bottle of beer and his untouched, curled-up sandwiches.

Neither of us said much on the return journey. For the old man's sake, I would try to resurrect the incubators, but seeing his rearing shed had given me the idea of how to cut out the work involved in duck rearing. Even if his incubators did not live on, his rearing method would.

I tried to put some of this into words, but Leslie cut me short. 'That's why I took you over,' he said. 'I'll go back and see him in a day or two, and give him a progress report. He'll die happier now.'

It became a point of honour to get those two old incubators working. During the journey home, two of the legs had fallen off one of them. There was no prospect of fixing them back on; the wood was too rotten and worm-eaten to hold any form of nail or screw. But two old orange boxes were exactly the right height, and also took the weight of the paraffin tank.

The pair were set up in the back kitchen, hoovered and painted with woodworm killer. Leslie showed me how to

135

trim the wick and adjust the old ether capsule thermostat. We filled them up with paraffin, lit the wick and, as it was by now very late, retired to bed, leaving the temperature adjustment till morning.

In the morning, we awoke to a smell of sooty paraffin pervading the whole house. Mercifully, I had shut the door into the back kitchen, which had kept most of the trouble in there. The paraffin tank on the orange boxes had leaked its entire contents onto the floor, and its flame had gone out. The other flame was galloping away, and clouds of black soot were spouting out of its chimney. The ceiling, the walls, the washing machine and all the week's washing, both done and waiting to be done, were covered with it. It was a miracle that we had not burned the house down.

I extinguished the sooty flame, shut the door again and said to my good lady wife, who was not so quietly having hysterics in the background, 'Please don't touch it. I'll clean it up when I come home from work this evening.'

The atmosphere was still distinctly chilly that evening, as well as stinking of soot and paraffin. She had spent all day trying to clean it up, and not really succeeding. 'They are going out,' she said, pointing at my incubators. 'They can go in that old shed up the back, and you can stink that out and burn it down to your heart's content.'

I could do little but acquiesce, and set about moving them up to the top of the yard. In the course of the move, I, too, became covered in oily soot, and broke one of the legs of the previously intact machine.

We replaced the leaking paraffin tank with another, retrimmed the wicks and tried again. This time we had two stinking smoking machines instead of one. At the height of it Leslie came up the drive. His trailer was overflowing with automatic water pots, food hoppers and infra-red lights.

'If I may make a suggestion,' he said, 'I have been to see my friend again, and he sends you these, with his compliments. He also said that the incubators tend to smoke if you use last year's wicks.' He went to his car and produced an old cardboard box, covered in dust and cobwebs. Inside it were enough new wicks to last us ten years.

We turned off the smoking monsters, rearranged the orange boxes to give the paraffin a more stable base and inserted the new wicks.

About three days and innumerable adjustments later, the machines were deemed stable enough in all respects to risk a few eggs in them.

Playing safe, we gathered up all the bantam eggs currently under hens, and gave the hens duck eggs to sit on. It relieved the hen crisis quite considerably, but did not lessen the work. The broodies still needed seeing to, and the eggs in the incubators needed turning three times a day.

*　　*　　*

By tacit agreement, I saw to the incubators. It took almost as long as if the eggs had been under broody hens—filling up the paraffin, trimming the wicks, adjusting the temperature and turning and moistening the eggs.

My wife looked after the broody hens. I had remarked to Leslie one evening that she was the best broody hen we had, and although it was a joke, it was substantially true. No matter how alike they may look to a mere male, each hen is an individual and needs an understanding of its own personal idiosyncrasies to get it to give of its best.

The scientist who gained immortality by coining the phrase 'peck order' when describing the behaviour of a flock of hens, was only telling the world what every farmer's wife has known since the first domestication of the fowl. Every flock has its boss hen whom nobody pecks back at. Number two pecks all except number one, and so on down the scale to the poor devil at the bottom who is pecked by everyone but cannot peck anybody back.

Our broody shed had thirty or forty sitting birds in it. Each one had its own nest in an orange box, with a sack over the entrance, held in place by two bricks. Once a day they were let off to feed and empty their bowels. The sack was necessary, since if one bird came off in its own time, there was no guarantee that it would go back to its own

137

nest, and if it chose the nest of a bird lower down the peck order, it could drive this hen off its nest and start a chain reaction. This had happened once, giving us half a shedful of cold and lifeless eggs. After their feed, they were all securely locked in the dark until the following day.

The hens that had been sitting in the shed longest were the natural bosses and, with their own established peck order, quietly got on with the business of feeding and ablution, when released together. If a newcomer was released with them, she was instantly attacked, to subjugate her to her proper station in life. None of them fed or cleansed themselves in the allotted time before the eggs got chilled, with the end result of fouled nests, restless hens, and bad temper all round.

Knowing every hen as an individual, Ruth released them in compatible batches of a half dozen or so at a time, and then, when they had had their statutory ten or twenty minutes off the nest, guided them back on it. There was an air of calm maternity in the broody shed, but it did take at least a couple of hours every day to see to them all.

I could never remember which boxes held compatible hens, so tended to release them in mathematical blocks— for example, all the hens against one wall together—and let them get on with it. By the time I was ready to put them back on the nests, the shed was a maelstrom of flying feathers, frantic hens and me chasing them round to get them back on a nest—any nest—before all my eggs got cold.

One never-to-be-forgotten day, Ruth had gone to see her parents and I was in sole charge. Thinking to save time, as I only had half an hour before my evening surgery, I let the lot off at once and opened the shed door so that they had more space to find some peace to feed in. I spent the first half hour of my surgery chasing panicking hens round the garden with a landing net, trying to catch them to put them back on their nests—a performance not guaranteed to bring the peace and harmony so necessary for a good hatch. At least half the hens showed every sign of having been forcibly jerked out of the broody state, as I left them standing, but imprisoned in their boxes, cackling their heads off in indignation.

After this fiasco, I threatened to adopt the standard method of the gamekeeper, who ties each hen by a piece of string on its leg to a peg in the ground. Each hen has its own food and water pot, and the string is too short to let it molest the hen next door. Apparently, once the hens get used to it, it works well, but on the occasion that I tried it with a particularly troublesome hen, she made so much fuss that I was forbidden to experiment further and almost banned from my own broody shed.

The mechanics of incubators I could understand. The psychology of hens was beyond me.

*　　*　　*

To everyone's delighted amazement, the first few clutches of bantams' eggs that had spent their last week in the incubators hatched magnificently. We could not spare hens to put them under, so I rigged up a temporary cardboard enclosure under one of the infra-red bulbs, and one of the old man's automatic drinkers, together with a food pot. After a few initial difficulties with the plumbing that either soaked or flooded everything, the system was declared ready to test and the chickens put in it.

They thrived and loved it. After about a week, however, they had grown enough feathers on their wings to fly out of the warm enclosure, but had not got enough sense to fly back in when they became cold. Almost as much time was spent catching and putting back the chicks as would have been spent moving coops and runs. The other problem not encountered before was cleaning out. A run that is moved every day leaves the mess behind. A batch of birds confined to one spot in a shed produces an incredible amount of droppings, not entirely mopped up by the continuing supply of sawdust and wood shavings provided.

But the experiment was deemed to have worked. More and more temporary sources of heat and water were hooked up somehow, and a satisfying flow of ducks emerged from the production line.

After a hen had killed every one of a particularly valuable clutch of ducklings as they hatched beneath her, we

139

put all the eggs near to hatch into the incubators and gave the hens the fresh eggs to start them off. When we reckoned that a hen had sat long enough in the shed, we gave her a clutch of incubator ducklings to rear, as a consolation prize. Those that we did not trust went back into the hen run.

Even so, we could have done with many more hens, and as the artificial method seemed to be just as good, more and more ducks went under the lights out of preference, rather than necessity.

At about two weeks old, the ducklings no longer needed extra heat, so were moved from the shed to small wire-netting enclosures outside, with a small plastic pond and a piece of old corrugated iron sheet on two straw bales for shelter. We had more ducks than we had ponds and shelters, so, after another week or two, they were released into a large communal enclosure, with a single bigger plastic pond, and no shelter. They all seemed to thrive, so much so that we put those ducks with hens attached in as well. The ducks loved it, but although some of the hens behaved impeccably, some of them seemed determined to kill every duckling that was not theirs. As all the ducks spent most of the time on the pond, the hens ran round and round it, pecking viciously at everything as they passed. In the end, we caught every hen and threw them all back into the hen run, where they seemed much more contented and infinitely less trouble.

All this automation seemed to bring much more, not less work for me, cleaning out sheds and ponds. But at least the burden on my wife was less; she now had some time to provide clean clothes and hot food.

Surveying it all one evening, after he had generously given me a hand with the nightly clean-up, Leslie said, 'If I may make a suggestion. All those derelict pigsties of yours—put a new roof on the old outside runs, and put the small ponds on a wire mesh, over a drain. It will be a lot less work, and you'll only need to clean out between batches.'

'Suggestion adopted,' I replied.

New roofs and drains cost money. I dared not even go

140

into the bank to face the unsympathetic deputy, let alone write a cheque for that amount. The improvements would have to wait until next year, paid for by the army of youngsters rapidly growing up.

Our friendly bank manager was keeping up his steady improvement when I paid him a routine visit. He was still in bed, but now only a delicate shade of lemon yellow, instead of the previous dark tan. He was sitting up, taking nourishment, and I hoped that he no longer had the proverbial jaundiced view of life, as I prepared to answer his question as to how the ducks were doing. I was taking a sample of blood from his arm at the time.

I explained to him how we had cut out a lot of the work, and told him about Leslie's suggestion for taking it further.

'That sounds all right to me,' he said, 'I'm sure the bank will have no qualms about financing that.'

'But what about your deputy?' I replied. 'He seems to be after my blood at the moment. I've just begged him not to close on us till I have sold the young ducks to the dealer. What's he going to say when I start putting up new roofs, drains and things?'

'It's like this,' he said. 'An established manager has a certain latitude with customers he knows personally. A deputy must go by the book and not acquire a single bad debt in his tenure of office. The book says that every person with an overdraft above the nominal figure must be sent a letter each week, asking for action. I should have sent you a letter three weeks out of every four for the past two years. If you promise to reduce that overdraft substantially over the next few months when you sell the ducks, I'll have a word with my deputy to give you an extension of credit.'

The world seemed a happier place as I left him, to take his sample of blood to the path lab. I had a financial reprieve, I knew a couple of chaps who would put up the roof and do the drains for the cost of the materials and their labour, and the number of ducks in the pens was increasing daily. There was not a single undiagnosed belly ache in the whole of the practice.

I 'phoned the duck dealer to come and collect some of the

older ones, as we were getting a bit overcrowded and I thought that they were ready.

To my surprise, he came the next day and inspected everything. He liked our ducks; they were good, he said, fat and healthy. But he did not like our automation that had produced them. He was a broody hen man, first and last.

After his tour of inspection, and when he had deftly captured all that were old enough to go, I tentatively raised the subject of payment.

'It won't be a lot, I'm afraid,' he said. 'You see, we still have last year's account and, if you'll forgive me, these are all the wrong sort of ducks.'

'What do you mean, the wrong sort of ducks?' I said indignantly.

'You know, the cheaper, commoner ones,' he replied. 'If you really want to make money, you need to breed the rarer and more expensive sorts.' He looked a bit thoughtful. 'And, besides, you haven't got any geese.'

Money did not change hands on that occasion.

Every few weeks after that he called and took away another consignment of ducks. When he arrived to collect the last few of the season, he came in an old van. Inside it were ducks that I had only dreamed of owning, and dozens of pairs of geese.

'I didn't have time to 'phone you, but I have just come from someone who has had to dispose of his birds. They're nearly all established breeding pairs, I've had his birds for years. I assumed you'd want them.'

'Well, yes,' I replied, as I watched him unload them and found myself carrying boxes down to the island. They were beautiful birds and, yes, I wanted them.

We loaded up the last of the home-bred birds, and went into the kitchen to settle up. After all the accounting was done, I still owed him a small sum of money. 'We'll put that on the account for next year,' he said. 'In this business, there is always next year.'

Ruth was fetching the children from school, so he did not stop long and had gone by the time she returned. Excitedly, I took them all down to the island to see my new

142

acquisitions.

'What about the money?' she said, 'How much has a whole summer of work come to, after allowance for your new birds?'

'We owe him ten pounds,' I said lamely, 'on the account for next year.' Then the realisation hit me. 'Whatever am I going to say to the bank? However can I tell them that he didn't pay us in money, he paid us in geese?'

Ah, well, there was always next year.

13

Every old house has its own particular ghost, and ours was no exception.

When we first went to look over the place, the children had rushed up into the attic rooms and declared with delight that here was the place to find ghosts.

The attic rooms were three in number, all with sloping roofs and ceilings and large dormer windows looking out over the tiles. The biggest room contained a full-size billiard table.

'That is included, of course,' said the owner. 'It would cost far too much to move it. As far as I know, it's been here since the major renovations in 1895. It must have been put in while they were doing the alterations, because there is no way it could come either in or out now.'

The boys stood on tip-toe and peered at us over the edge as they contemplated its enormity. It was just too big for them.

'Are there any ghosts in this house?' John asked irrelevantly.

The owner looked at him, as if composing an answer that would not frighten him.

Oh, God, I thought, please say 'no'.

'If there are, this is the room they'll be in,' John continued happily. 'I can feel that this is the ghostly room.'

The owner evaded the question by remaining silent but caught my eye. There obviously were ghosts.

The boys found the rack of billiard cues and eyed them hopefully.

'Can we have a go?' they pleaded. I looked at the owner.

'Please,' said all three boys together.

The owner looked back at me. 'It's your table,' he said, and that was when I first realised that he had already sold the place to me.

Armed with billiard cues longer than themselves, and

144

with chins just clearing the top of the table, they began to play a sort of hockey with the cues and balls.

'Hang on a minute,' I admonished them, 'you'll break everything. Let me show you the proper way.'

Games without Father showing them the proper way were always much more fun.

'Are there ghosts here?' John repeated.

The owner was ready this time. 'Only friendly ones,' he said nonchalantly.

This seemed to satisfy John's curiosity and, proper billiards being much less entertaining than improvised hockey, we covered the table up again and went downstairs.

The ghosts, friendly or otherwise, had not bothered us. Ancient boards creaked in the night, and the back door continually slipped its latch and blew open a few inches. When it did so the wind, from even a minor breeze, howled through the crack in a very mournful and irritating manner, but nobody ever associated either natural phenomenon with ghostly origins.

The house was too full of people and life—that is, until Ruth took the family for a holiday with her parents for a couple of weeks, leaving me to cope with the ducks and work on my own.

* * *

Early one morning, after they had gone, I locked up the house and set off to the surgery, as normal. It was not until I came home that evening and suffered the solitude of a lonely supper and an empty evening stretching uninvitingly ahead, that I realised how big and how eerie an old house could be. Each new gust of wind, and each fresh creak in the floor-boards really startled me, so that I began to imagine all sorts of things. Several times, in spite of myself, I had to go all over the house and check that no burglar had come in uninvited, and that no fox or other predator had got in among my ducks. When the telephone rang, the loud jangle shattered my nervous system, so that I literally leaped a foot in the air before I answered it.

It was only the hospital telephonist, with whom I had made an arrangement that, if I had to go out, she would take all my calls for me during my absence, confirming that she was now on duty. During that whole evening, I did not once have to go out, and it was one of the worst evenings of my life. Going up to bed and lying alone in that great big bed, in that great big room, while the creaks and groans carried on relentlessly, did not induce a suitable state of mind for untroubled sleep. Nor did a couple of owls, hooting miserably at each other in the trees just outside my room, improve my slumber.

At this stage I did not think of ghosts, not even when, in the middle of the night, I did have to go out, returning more alone and miserable than ever.

The second night was even worse than the first. I had come home late, tired and hungry. Of course there was no supper ready, I would have to get my own; but I had completely forgotten about this. It was theoretically a night not on call, so, armed with a stiff drink and the frying pan, I set about cooking myself a simple meal.

Several drinks later and with a stomach not only full, but positively uncomfortable, I prepared for bed. The various noises off were distinctly un-nerving. Several times I quite convinced myself that there was somebody else moving around the house and, on one of my trips upstairs to check the empty bedrooms, I was quite sure that I could hear the click of billiard balls and the sound of feet walking round the table. It took considerable courage, and another stiff drink, to get me up to the billiard room.

I switched on the light, flinging open the door as I did so.

The room was silent and empty, the cloth on the table undisturbed. As I switched off the light and closed the door again, there was quite definitely the sound of creaking boards, as if someone were walking round the room. Maintaining dignity and forcing myself to walk slowly, I fled. I only partially believed that it was the ancient boards straightening themselves, after the passage of my own feet.

When I was back in the safety of the kitchen and reaching for yet another tot of comfort from the bottle, the back

146

door slipped its latch, swung half open, and a cold blast of air entered, moaning through the cracks.

The realisation that there was nobody the other side of the door was probably more of a shock than the door opening spontaneously in the first place.

The awful wind noise stopped as I slammed the door and locked it. In the silence that followed, I could hear the ducks quacking and muttering complaints, and I realised that they were demanding food. I had forgotten to feed them.

Swearing, I put on my boots and coat and set off. It was a clear, dark night, with great patches of heavy cloud moving fairly rapidly across the sky. Between the patches of moving cloud, the moon lit up the garden and island with a silvery, colourless light that suddenly went out, as the moon passed behind a cloud.

With a sack of food on my back and my nerves in shreds from my over-active imagination, I was not exactly prepared to meet anyone else wandering round the garden, but as I walked down to the ducks' enclosure, I realised that there was somebody standing by the gate.

It was an old man, dressed in a tatty overcoat and battered trilby hat. He stood there, totally silent, swaying gently backwards and forwards.

I stopped walking and stood there looking at him, half expecting him to move, or speak, or do something, and half trying to make myself call out to him. I was aware of the weight of the sack of food on my back.

Undecided whether to ask him what the hell he was doing there, or whether to be more sociable, I suddenly realised that I could see right through him, to the island and field beyond.

Standing immobile, with half a hundredweight of duck food on one's back, is not the best position from which to take sudden flight. In all honesty, I was rooted to the spot, frozen in terror.

As my wits returned, I realised that I had three choices: to continue standing there, to drop the sack and run, or to keep walking towards him and go and feed those hungry ducks.

147

The ducks were singularly unperturbed by my dilemma. They had heard and seen me coming, and were quacking and clammering a greeting to their food.

Perhaps it was their very normality in the face of a transparent old man, a real live ghost—if there was such a thing—that eventually persuaded me to keep on walking.

'Good evening,' I called out to him—more a shout to encourage myself than a greeting.

At the unexpected sound of my voice, all the ducks went silent. The old man continued to sway gently back and forth. I could feel my heart pounding as I walked towards him.

Just as I was on the point of dropping the sack and running, the ducks started quacking again. I knew that if I ran, I would not be able to go back alone inside that creaking house, with its self-opening door and moaning wind noises. The only place I could run to was the car, and where could I go then? I should feel such a fool telling anybody that I had run away from home, from a ghost.

As I walked towards my ghost, concentrating on the field I could see through him, the moon went behind a small cloud for a few seconds, and as the light diminished, the old man disappeared.

With pounding heart, I walked on to where he had been.

I know now why fright can give people heart attacks, I thought stupidly.

The moon reappeared from behind its cloud, and so did the old man, only this time he was not a real but transparent, ghostly old man, but moonlight shining on the wire-netting fence, in the shape of an old man wearing an old overcoat and a trilby hat.

The moonlight was shining through the trees onto the fence. In the shadow of the trees the fence was invisible, but in the moonlight the fence glowed translucently in that ghostly shape. The movement was caused by the swaying branches of the trees and the rhythmic rocking of the wire-netting in the wind.

Thank goodness I didn't run, I said to myself, as I tipped the food into the empty hoppers and the ducks scrabbled round me eating it. It seemed so lovely and peaceful, on a lakeside in the moonlight, listening to the sounds of water-fowl and the other myriad noises of the night.

I went back up the garden, and from the same position reviewed my ghost. The moon had gone behind a cloud, and my ghost had gone. I waited for a few moments, but he did not reappear. Even when the moon came out again, it had moved relative to the trees, and the light shining on the netting no longer bore even the remotest resemblance to my old man.

Inside the house, the creaks and groans continued, but now somehow subtly changed. They, too, were no longer fearsome, suggestive of intruders; they were the friendly, comforting sounds of normality. I no longer felt alone.

The owner had been right. If there were ghosts in this old house, they were friendly ones.

The remainder of the two weeks on my own passed very peacefully. I was alone, but not lonely. The family returned and the house was full of noise and movement again. Ruth and I had laughed over the telephone, when I had told her of how much I had frightened myself with moonlit wire-netting, but now, in the excitement of their homecoming, neither of us thought to tell the children about it, or anyone else, for that matter. The incident faded into memory and was temporarily forgotten.

*　　*　　*

It was recalled from memory very abruptly one evening some months later.

We were converting the old pigsties into duck rearing sheds, following Leslie Warner's suggestion. These pigsties were of the old-fashioned sort: a row of five comfortable back rooms, each with a small open yard in front, the whole built solidly of brick.

Our conversion was merely to add a tin roof to the open yards, and fence in the sides with mouse-proof wire-netting. It gave us a lovely warm room at the back, which, when equipped with infra-red heaters and automatic water pots, provided ideal accommodation for broods of small ducks as they hatched. As the ducks grew, merely by

149

opening the door they could be allowed into the front yard, where they could make as much mess as they liked.

There is no doubt that ducks *are* messy things. Water is for jumping in, and for splashing about as far as possible. Our solution to the ever-increasing work of cleaning out soaked litter was to place the water pot over a drain covered with a piece of tough wire mesh. An automatic ball-cock valve kept the water pot full, and they could splash as much as they liked down into the drain.

There is a snag to most good ideas. The problem with this one was that water does not flow uphill and, when it does flow, it collects somewhere. The water pots had to be raised up in the air, and the ducks given access to them by massive concrete ramps. From here, rat-proof channels had to be constructed to a main drain and soak-away. Half the two-man gang who had erected the roofing had returned to help me with the concreting and digging.

This half of the gang suffered from indigestion, and his name was Benny. He worked as a jack-of-all-trades for a local builder. His indigestion was easy enough to cure with simple old-fashioned white mixtures, but it kept recurring. He was a regular attender at the surgery for yet another bottle, and when I pointed out to him that he could buy this stuff cheaply from the chemist, without the bother of taking time off work to come and see me, he was quite offended.

'Medicines should only be prescribed by doctors,' he said. 'I don't believe in all that muck you get from chemists.'

It transpired that he was a born worrier. On each visit, he needed reassurance that his malady was only simple indigestion. He worried about money—about not having enough, and about not getting enough overtime to earn it. He had jumped at the chance of several weeks of evening work erecting my duck sheds, and had brought his mate along to help him.

He reckoned that he could manage alone on the concreting and digging.

On the evening in question he was at the top of the yard, digging on his own. At least he was, until he came charging into the kitchen without even bothering to knock. Usually he tapped timidly on the door, poked his cap-covered head round it and enquired deferentially if he could come in.

He stood, white as a sheet, gasping for breath, and leaned with his hands on the kitchen table.

'Whatever's the matter?' I asked him, somewhat startled by his abrupt entry. 'Have you seen a ghost, or something?'

'Yes,' he said, as he sat uninvited at the table and began to shake violently. He looked imploringly at us, and beads of sweat began to form on his face. 'Can I have some brandy, please?'

I poured him half a tumblerful and watched him gulp it down. It restored the colour to his face, but I dreaded to think what it would do for his indigestion. He put down his glass and gave an almighty burp.

'Sorry for that,' he said somewhat shamefacedly, but he looked better.

'What happened?' I asked.

'Nothing, really,' he said, 'and that's the stupid part.' He looked earnestly first at Ruth and then at me. 'Did you know you had a ghost up there?'

'No,' I replied honestly, for I could not really call my moonlit wire-netting a proper ghost.

'Well, there is one,' he said emphatically. 'I've just seen it.'

We both sat down at the table. Ruth produced two more glasses, and he pushed his now empty one towards her for a refill.

'What sort of ghost was it?' she asked him softly.

Now that he had regained his composure, and with the best part of the second glass inside him, he settled down to tell us his tale. I could already visualise him, boring many a Saturday evening in the pub to death, with repetitions of it. But at least we were having the first, unedited version. He took a deep breath and began.

'Well, you know I was digging that trench up there?' looking again at us both for confirmation. 'I thought at first it was Leslie come looking for you. He just walked up the

151

yard, and stood by me, while I was spading it out. When he didn't say anything, I stopped and looked up at him. It wasn't Leslie, it was just an old bloke in a tatty old coat and a scruffy old trilby hat.' He paused. 'More like an old tramp, if you know what I mean.'

I knew what he meant. He was describing my ghost, but I was sure neither Ruth nor I had mentioned it to him.

'He just stood there looking at me,' he said.

A shiver ran up my spine. The room suddenly felt very cold. I reached for a refill of my glass, and two more were pushed towards the bottle.

'"Wotcher, mate," I said to him,' Benny continued, 'and he just stood there looking at me, swaying gently, like.' He took another drink of my brandy. 'And that was when I realised he didn't have any feet.'

'What do you mean, he didn't have any feet?' Ruth said disbelievingly.

'Just that,' Benny replied. 'His legs started half-way up.'

We both stared at him, not knowing whether to believe him or not.

'Then I saw that I could see through him.'

'What did you do then?' I asked, after a pause, for he seemed to have dried up.

'Damn' near messed my trousers,' he confessed.

'Were you looking down towards the island?' I asked, thinking that he might have seen the same moonlight as me.

'No,' he replied, somewhat puzzled. 'He was between me and the sheds. I could see the shed through him. One of the doors was open and swinging a bit. I could see it moving through his chest.'

'What happened then?' Ruth asked.

'He sort of faded away,' he said lamely, 'and as soon as he'd gone, I got the hell out of it and came in here.'

We sat silently at the table for a while.

'Shall we all go up there now, and see if he's still there?' I said eventually.

'No,' Benny replied with some feeling. 'If you don't mind, I'm going to pack up now and go home. I'll leave all my tools where they are and bring my mate back with me

152

tomorrow to finish it off in daylight. I don't want to go back up there on my own again, not in the dark.'

After he'd gone, Ruth asked, 'Do you really think he saw a ghost?'

'I don't know,' I replied, 'but Benny will believe to his dying day that he did.'

We did walk up the yard, with all available lights on, and each with a powerful torch.

All there was up there was a half-dug trench, and a spade.

It was several days before Benny came back with his mate, on a Saturday afternoon, in daylight. He would never go up there alone in the dark again.

After this incident, which we deliberately did not repeat to the children in case it frightened them, we tended to forget all about ghosts.

They, however, did not forget about us.

*　　*　　*

Ever since we had moved, several of our friends had been coming sporadically to spend an evening on the billiard table, and a sort of Thursday evening club had developed. They took it in turns to bring the beer, and a few pence changed hands on the outcome of each game. The boys loved to come up and join us for the precious moments before they were packed off to bed. They would cadge a few furtive sips of beer and advise knowingly on how each shot should be played.

Tom had joined us for the first time that night. He was a neighbouring farmer who specialised in onion growing; I was reliably informed that what he did not know about onions was not worth knowing. He was a stocky, black-haired man, exceedingly handsome, and although he was now respectably married with a family similar to our own, still had the reputation of his youth, of being very much a ladies' man.

He had come with Peter, the policeman, who, determined that he was not going to lose his few pence yet again, had boasted that he would bring as his partner the

153

local snooker champion. Tom, of course, had not been informed of this, and thought that he had merely come for the beer. His standard of play was, however, considerably better than our usual.

Young John took an instant liking to him and adopted him as his champion, helping him to drink his beer and giving him very profound advice on the lie of the snooker balls. The evening was going well; they were scoring ten points to our one.

Tom lined up to play a particularly beautiful shot. If he potted this ball, the rest of the table was wide open for a big break, and his and the policeman's five pence were assured. He bent over the table and looked down his cue. John, standing right beside him, continued to give helpful advice directly into his ear.

He brought his cue back for the strike and, just as he brought it forward again to hit his ball, John whispered confidentially into his ear, 'We've got ghosts in this room. I've seen them.'

Tom's cue hit the ball somewhat harder than he had intended, so far off centre that it developed a vicious spin and shot off sideways like a golfer's slice. It hit the cushion with considerable force, jumped over it and fell with a loud bang onto the floor.

John was horrified. 'You've given them four points,' he said, as the rest of us collapsed in helpless laughter.

Tom stood up, looking distinctly pale. 'Yes,' he said, and began to gaze slowly and furtively round the room, as if he was looking for the ghosts that John had now forgotten after the catastrophe of his exceedingly foul shot.

The ball was retrieved and replaced on the table and, amid many ribald comments about ghostly hands guiding the cue, the game continued.

John was most indignant. 'There *are* ghosts up here,' he insisted. 'We've all seen them,' and, addressing his two smaller brothers, 'haven't we?'

'Yes,' they said together, solemnly nodding their little heads in agreement.

'They're nice, friendly ghosts, though,' I hurriedly interrupted.

'Oh, yes,' they agreed nonchalantly.

At that moment Ruth shouted up the stairs, for the boys to come down for bath and bed, and reluctantly they left us. The game continued among much discussion as to what the boys had really seen, and what they had imagined, but Tom was barely able to hit his ball, let alone score from it.

'Those ghosts have proper upset you, haven't they, partner?' Peter remarked, after Tom's third successive miss, and, turning to me, asked, '*Are* there ghosts up here?'

'I don't know,' I replied. 'If there are, I've never seen one, but the chap we bought the house from did remark that they were very friendly.'

Tom did not look at all happy, but did his best to grin and shrug it off. 'The only ghost I've ever seen wasn't very friendly,' he said, as he played yet another appalling shot, donating four more points to our score.

'You'd better tell us all about it, partner,' said Peter. 'You might play a bit better when you've got it off your chest.'

By mutual consent, we all put down our cues and retired to the makeshift bar at the end of the room, where Peter refilled the beer mugs.

Tom tipped his back in one swallow. Peter refilled it. 'Come on, partner,' he said, 'tell your uncle all about it. You'd better tell the truth, now, 'cos if you tell a lie, those ghosts up here might come out of the woodwork and spill your beer.'

We all laughed, and settled down to Tom's narrative.

Our house stands four-square, on a slight hill, facing due south. From the attic windows, the view over the countryside is superb, and right in the middle of the view is another small hill, about a mile away, which is completely covered with scrubby old trees—Devil's Wood.

It was completely dark outside, but Tom pointed out through the window, in the direction of Devil's Wood.

'It was all a long time ago,' he said, 'just after I'd left school and started working for my father.' He paused and took another swig of beer. 'We didn't know then that all those old mounds of earth in the wood were big graves.'

'I didn't know that there were graves in Devil's Wood,' I interrupted him.

'Oh, yes,' he continued. 'We looked it all up afterwards. The chap from Norwich Museum told us that there had been a lot of old battles round here, Saxons and Vikings and so on, and some Romans. Apparently there was one hell of a big one on the top of that hill there, and when it was all over, there were best part of a thousand bodies to bury. They just piled them in heaps, then covered them with earth.'

'Good God,' I said, 'I didn't know that.'

'Neither did we,' Tom said, 'when we went in to get those trees out.'

'What were you doing, getting trees out of Devil's Wood?' asked Peter curiously.

'Father had a big tractor,' he explained. 'The place belonged to Old Jones then, and he asked Father and me to give him a hand to drag the timber out. Most of it was easy, but one great big ugly brute got itself stuck on the side of a mound between several other trees, didn't it?'

He paused for effect. We waited for him to continue.

'Well,' he said at last, 'we'd got that trunk completely stuck, hadn't we? and it seemed that the only way we were going to get it out was to pull the other trees out by their roots and make some room for it. We put a chain round the biggest of them, hitched it to the winch and pulled.'

'Do you know,' he continued, as if expecting us not to believe him, 'the whole damn' lot came over together, didn't it? It took the top off that mound like taking the lid off a box, and all those old skeletons spilled out all over the place. Fair gave us a fright, I'll tell you.'

'Where does the ghost come in?' asked Peter casually, as he reached for another bottle of beer. 'Did they all leap up out of the grave, shouting ghostly Saxon slogans?'

'No, you fool,' Tom replied, as he took the bottle out of Peter's hand. 'You just be patient, and I'll tell you.'

He filled his glass and drank half of it.

'What did you do with all those skeletons?' I asked him.

'Put the damn' things back and covered 'em up again, quick,' he replied in a matter-of-fact voice. 'We knew they were old, as some of those trees growing on them must have been there for at least a couple of hundred years.'

'Didn't you tell anybody, the police for instance?' asked Peter.

'Old Jones rang up Norwich Museum. They told him that they knew all about them, and on no account was he to disturb them, so we covered them up and left them be.'

'What about the ghost?' Peter demanded again, but Tom ignored him, and continued with his story.

'We left that great ugly trunk half buried in the mound— it's still there, by the way, just where we left it—got the rest of the timber out, packed up and went home.'

He looked at Peter across the top of his now empty glass.

'I was sparking a girl out thataway,' he said, vaguely waving his arm at the window. 'Hadn't got a motor bike in those days, so I had to walk. The quickest way from my house to hers was over the fields, alongside Devil's Wood. Done the trip dozens of times, knew the path well.'

We could all sense that he was coming up to his ghost, and waited quietly for him to carry on.

'This particular night, I thought as how I'd go into the wood and have another look at all those skeletons. The museum had sent a chap out, and he'd told Old Jones all about the battles and things, and I must have been thinking about them. It must have been a hell of a fight, with a thousand dead, and all they'd got to kill each other with was swords and axes. I remember I was thinking that I'd dig out a bone or two, and see if there were any sword cuts, when the whole wood went deathly quiet and horribly cold, all of a sudden, like.'

He shivered visibly, shook it off, and passed his glass for a refill.

'It got quieter and quieter as I neared that mound, and I have never, before or since, felt so cold.'

He paused, and looked at us each in turn.

'I kept on walking,' he said quietly, 'only I noticed that the silence had stopped. There was a sort of moaning, like something in pain; it was all around me, I couldn't pinpoint where it was coming from, and I couldn't tell exactly when it had started. I had to keep stopping, to try to find

157

out, but I couldn't.'

He paused again, holding the full glass untouched in his hand.

'I didn't see it at first.' he said. 'One minute there was just this great big ugly tree trunk sticking out of the side of that mound, and then, when I looked again, there was this bloody-great big, angry Viking standing on it, waving his sword at me, wasn't there?'

'You're having us on,' Peter said, after a few moments.

'As true as I'm standing here, I'm not,' he replied. 'I can still see him now, sort of silvery, like a black and white photograph, waving that sword at me. The expression on his face was evil, pure evil, under that cow-horn helmet, and hair sticking out all over the place.' The full glass in his hand trembled slightly. 'He'd got a sort of short skirt on, with baggy trousers underneath, tied on with criss-cross ribbons up his legs, and he looked as if he was coming straight for me.'

Tom stopped speaking and stared challengingly at me.

'Did he come for you?' I asked. Though far-fetched, the manner in which Tom was telling his story seemed real enough for it to be true.

'Didn't stop to find out,' he replied, and began to drink his beer.'

'What did you do, then?' asked Peter.

'Got a date, hadn't I?' he said, as he put down the glass. 'Kept it, of course.'

Peter stared at him. 'Didn't you run, or anything?'

'Course I damn' well did. Faster than you could. Every time I ran into some twigs, I thought he'd got me, and if I looked out for twigs, I tripped over the roots and frightened the pants off myself.'

'Did he follow you out of the wood, then?'

'Didn't stop to see. I just kept going.'

'Then what happened?'

'Well, I got to this girl's house, all of a sweat and a lather, and frightened out of my wits. Her parents were out, so she sort of comforted me on the sofa, like, and made me feel better.'

'You damn' fool, Tom,' Peter muttered scathingly. 'You

158

don't expect us to believe that, do you?'

'You can believe what you like,' he replied evenly, 'but you can take it from me, when you've had the pants frightened off you, like I had, there's nothing quite like a nice warm, loving woman to bring things back to normality.'

'More likely it was she who took the pants off you, the ghost had nothing to do with it,' Peter remarked with a mixture of scorn and disbelief, 'and that's your excuse for being found running trouserless down the road, with her father after you.'

We all laughed, but Tom continued, slightly put out that we did not seem wholly to believe him. 'No, honestly, Doc,' he said looking straight at me, 'it's a fact, I was scared stupid when I got there, and after about an hour, I felt that I must have imagined the whole thing.'

I nodded agreement at him.

'Well,' he continued. 'when I left her later that night, it seemed daft to go all the long way home round the road, so I took my usual short cut back across the fields, up by the edge of Devil's Wood.'

'Did you see it again?' Peter interrupted.

'I don't know,' Tom replied, half serious. 'When I started off, it seemed daft to be scared of going past that wood, and I shouldn't be going anywhere near that mound, but the nearer I got to it, the more scared I got, didn't I?' He paused for a few moments. 'I came past that wood on tiptoe, looking for it, and getting myself into a hell of a state.'

He paused again. 'You know that dip in the path, just past those old beech trees? Well, I'd just got to there, and thought I was safe, when I trod on this thing.'

He looked me full in the face. 'I thought I'd been frightened before, but blast me, it was nothing to this. You know the four-minute mile? That bloke only thinks he holds the record, really it's mine. It's about a mile from there home, and, Doc, I did it in less than a minute that night.'

'What was it you trod on?' I asked unnecessarily.

'One of Old Jones' pigs. It must have got out, and was fast asleep on that path. I stood right in the middle of it. I can remember feeling how soft and squelchy it was, before it moved and squealed enough to move all the bats out of

159

hell.' He paused again. 'Doc, I didn't know I could run so fast.'

'If you ran that fast,' Peter said, 'how did you know it was a pig you tripped over?'

'I don't,' said Tom, after a moment. 'But if it wasn't a pig, what the hell was it? The only thing it could possibly have been was one of Old Jones' pigs. If it wasn't, I've *felt* a ghost, as well as seen one.'

None of us knew whether to believe him or not, and Peter said so.

'Please yourself,' Tom replied. 'I'm not bothered whether you do or don't, but I know what I saw, and every time anybody talks about ghosts, it sets me all on edge for a while.'

He walked away from the bar and picked up his cue. 'Come on,' he said, as he bent over the table. 'I've got it off my chest. Now let's finish this game.'

The play was desultory and uninspired, and did not last long. We finished it, replaced the cloth on the table and retired down to the kitchen for a final cup of coffee before they all went home. There was no more talk of ghosts.

As I showed them all out of the back door and walked into the yard to the assembled cars, I glanced up to the top of the yard, thinking that I had seen our own ghostly old man again, but on close inspection there was nothing there.

'Who was that?' asked Tom.

'Where?' I said.

'That old tramp up the yard,' he replied.

'Oh, him,' I said. 'Only our resident ghost. He's harmless.' But I was talking to myself. They had all leapt into their cars and were rapidly departing.

14

Mrs Johnson was such a nice motherly body. Round and comfortable, in her grey check coat and neat, blue-rinsed white hair, she reminded me of our female emperor goose. She had the same habit of cocking her head on one side while she jabbered soft-voiced nothings at the world in general.

After I had examined her, she levered herself up off the couch and stood by the side of it, naked. She and the goose had exactly the same shaped abdomen, and the same little spindly legs set well back, wide apart.

When once again girt in her corsets and covered by her well-fitting coat, even her walk had the same well-meaning maternal waddle. Again, like the goose, she suffered from arthritis of the joints, and a form of muscular rheumatism. The goose I could do nothing about, but Mrs Johnson I could and had, relieving her symptoms considerably.

*   *   *

The goose that Mrs Johnson so resembled had been acquired from the duck dealer, together with her aged mate, for a very nominal sum, on the basis that they were both well past breeding age and needed a good retirement home. They had settled in immediately and remained completely trusting and friendly. Merely to walk down to the island was the signal for them to heave themselves arthritically from their usual resting place and amble towards us. Having reached us, they would chatter softly to us and to each other, as they waited for the inevitable slice of bread. They nibbled at it delicately, together, talking ceaselessly. All the time that we stayed there, the geese accompanied us, waddling amiably behind, keeping up their running commentary.

Come nesting time, they built themselves a cosy heap of vegetation, into which she deposited three eggs. Emmy, as we called her, to distinguish her from her husband, Uncle Fred, did not appear to leave the nest at all, not even to feed, and we seriously doubted whether she would have the strength to survive the incubation period, or, if she came through, whether her arthritic legs would ever work again after all that time sitting down.

Several times I approached the nest, with the express intention of picking up her eggs and hatching them in the incubator, but on each occasion came away empty handed. I took her some food instead, which she ate daintily and confidingly from my hand, while Uncle Fred expressed grave concern and fussed around her.

One morning, those three eggs had hatched. Three little grey heads peeped out from under her breast feathers, nattering just like their mother in high-pitched voices. Uncle Fred sat beside them, nattering back. He rose stiffly to meet me as I approached and, expressing little aggression, but much pride and concern, allowed me to handle them. Emmy made no attempt to leave the nest, but ate greedily out of my hand. The little ones nibbled inquisitively at my fingers.

I left them there and went off to work. At lunch time they were still there, and we feared that Emmy was unable to stand, having made absolutely no attempt to do so. I fed them again.

That evening they were still there and, fearing that they were too vulnerable down on the island, we decided to move them to a small enclosure on the lawn. With a goose under each arm, and the goslings sitting in the food bucket, I carried them up to the house. Throughout the journey, the entire family went on nattering to each other, apparently utterly unconcerned by the move. I put them down on the lawn, gave them a food and water pot, and stood back to watch what happened. If there was the slightest hint that Uncle Fred and Emmy were incapable of looking after the goslings properly, they would have to go into one of the sheds, under a light, and be reared with the ducks.

Emmy rose creakily to her feet and tottered to the water pot, where she had an obviously very refreshing drink. The little ones followed her and nibbled at it. Uncle Fred, without a care in the world, set about the food. We left them, some time later, sitting side by side, muttering sweet nothings to each other, while the goslings burrowed under her breast.

They made perfect and very proud parents. It was almost possible to see those goslings grow, and after a few days we gave them the freedom of the front lawn. They were never as confiding as their parents, tending to hang behind them, and backing off if we approached too close, especially after a visit from the duck dealer, when they had been unceremoniously upended to expose the more intimate parts of their anatomy, and pronounced to be three females.

We decided to keep them all, and ordered from the duck dealer three young and handsome ganders to form the nucleus of the new breeding flock.

*   *   *

Watching Mrs Johnson walk across from the couch to the chair, and straining hard to catch what she was saying, I found myself thinking about the geese, and the way Emmy led her brood across the lawn.

Mrs Johnson had suffered for years from a condition called polymyalgia rheumatica, an inflammation of the muscles that causes a very painful stiffness. It responds well to the cortisone-type drugs which, after a few months, can usually be tailed off, with complete relief of symptoms. In Mrs Johnson's case, however, every time that I tried to reduce the dose, her pain and stiffness recurred.

She had now developed another painful complaint, osteoporosis, a thinning and softening of the bones, particularly of the spine, causing the individual spinal bones to collapse. The process had probably been aggravated by the cortisone that she had taken for so long, but there was no question of stopping it. I should have to give her injections of another type of steroid hormone, to strengthen her bones. These injections were a variation of the male hormone, the treatment that Russian women athletes had been taking to build them up in order to throw Olympic missiles further. I did not like giving the two together, but there was no other way to ease her pain. I warned her that she would have to take them for several months before she got any significant relief, and showed her to the door.

During those months she slowly improved, and again any attempt to reduce the doses was followed by instant relapse. During those months, too, Emmy and Uncle Fred, with their brood of adolescent daughters, had been banished from the front lawn, back to the island, whither they were shooed with extreme reluctance on their part. The trio of eligible young bachelors duly arrived, and in spite of Uncle Fred's best, but somewhat elderly endeavours, his daughters preferred their company to his. He eventually accepted resignedly the new additions to his family and spent most of his time trying to get them to shape up to his standards of behaviour.

Early in the New Year, Mrs Johnson came for one of her routine checks, and confided diffidently to me that she had 'a little touch of women's problem'. This, of course, was after she had dressed again following the examination, so we had to start all over again and look at the gynaecological department. It was a simple hormone deficiency problem, that should be easily cured by giving her a course of female hormone.

In view of the fact that she was already taking two other hormones, I consulted our local gynaecologist before giving them to her.

'Should be no problem,' he boomed down the phone at me, in his usual extrovert and flower-in-his-button-hole voice. 'Sometimes increases the libido a bit, but that shouldn't be any problem. Does 'em good. Husbands like it.' So after establishing the dose, I prescribed them.

They did indeed increase her libido; she positively bloomed. Compared to her, poor old Emmy looked distinctly decrepit. Once again any attempt by me to reduce the doses was met with gentle, but definite opposition.

164

She looked and felt so well that it was hard to deny her.

With the coming of spring, the ducks and geese started their usual courtship displays, and the geese started fighting for territory. Uncle Fred and Emmy seemed very gentle and confiding, but not very active. Once or twice I watched them half-heartedly attempt to mate, but Fred did not seem to have his mind on it, and Emmy looked relieved.

Sitting thinking about them in the surgery one evening, a thought probably provoked by the next name on my appointment list, Mrs Johnson, I pressed the bell to call her in. A little mousy man entered, dignified and gentle. He walked into the room as if he was carrying a heavy load on his shoulders, his back bent and his knees shaking.

I motioned him to the chair, into which he sank gratefully. He gazed at me with sad, tired eyes, and his little grey moustache, that ought to have been a spritely toothbrush, drooped in deep melancholy.

'I've come about my wife,' he said.

I picked up the records. 'Mrs Johnson? Mrs Emily Johnson?'

'That's her. I'm Fred Johnson. I'm not sure whether it's me or her I want to see you about.' Diffidently he searched for words.

'Tell me all about it,' I prompted him. 'She seemed so well last time she came.'

'That's exactly the problem,' he murmured softly. 'I don't know whether she's been ill all these years and is now better, or whether it's just me getting old, or perhaps ill myself. But I don't feel ill, just tired. Too tired to cope with anything any more.'

I sat, and waited for the narrative to continue. He dropped his eyes and sat hunched, clasping his hands together, staring at the floor. It was obviously very embarrassing for him to talk about it. I wondered if it had something to do with his wife's newly developed increase of libido.

I waited. Eventually he looked up at me, waved his hands dejectedly in the air and then resignedly placed them on his knees.

'We've been married thirty years,' he pleaded. 'I think

165

they've been happy,' and lapsed into silence again. I could feel him searching for the words to express his feelings.

'It's not natural.' He paused. 'At our time of life,' and tailed off into a longer pause.

'You see,' he started again, still looking at the floor, 'I, er, we, er, our life in bed was never anything exciting. We enjoyed it after we were first married, but after the children were born it sort of settled into a routine. Necessity, if you see what I mean, like being constipated. You don't feel well if you don't go. I, er, didn't feel well if I didn't, er, go.'

He looked up at me, and I nodded encouragement at him.

'It.' He lapsed into silence again. 'We.' He changed his mind and started again. 'She was always afraid of getting pregnant again, after the second child, so I never went all the way. You know, like you were taking the train to Lowestoft, and got off at Oulton Broad.'

'I know,' I said. 'Withdrawal. It's the oldest contraceptive method in the book. Didn't you ever use any other method?'

He shook his head. 'At first, I tried to buy some from a chemist, but each time that I went into his shop, his young lady assistant came to serve me, and I just couldn't ask her. So I bought a tube of toothpaste, and after about the seventh tube of toothpaste, I just didn't bother. It didn't seem to matter. We just carried on as before and, you know, we just didn't seem to need it so often. Just occasionally, you know, like Christmas, or a birthday treat. And then she got this rheumatism, and it all came to a stop.'

He came to a stop as well; the flood of words had exhausted him. After a little while he continued. 'Well, since you've been treating her rheumatism, she's been so much better, and since we both know she won't get pregnant now, we sort of started again.'

Another pause. 'Really, *she* started again. It was always me who got things going, but now it's her, and she makes me go all the way home on the train, if you know what I mean.'

He looked at me imploringly. 'You've got to do something about it, Doctor, I just can't keep it up. She wants it first thing in the morning, and when I come home for lunch, and again in bed at night.'

He was almost crying. 'I just can't satisfy her. I'm nearly on my knees. They've threatened me with the sack at work, if I don't pull my socks up. I just can't do it.' Those soulful, tired eyes were pleading with me. 'It'll kill me if I go on like this.'

Oh, God, I thought. What have I done? I shall just have to reduce his wife's hormone dosage, in spite of her protests.

To him I said, 'Pop on the couch, and I'll just check that it's not you.'

Wearily, he climbed up onto the couch. He had hardly the strength to lift his legs on. Not expecting to find anything, I barely noticed his extreme weakness and the dark patches of pigmentation where he should have been white. It was not until I took his blood pressure, which was exceedingly low, that the penny dropped. He had Addison's disease, failure of his adrenal glands. Whether this was pre-existing, or provoked by his wife's nymphomania, was a moot point, probably the latter.

With considerable relief, I told him of my provisional diagnosis, and sent him off to have the necessary blood tests to confirm it. Three days later he was back, and I waved the pathology reports at him in triumph. He looked dreadful and felt worse. I gave him a prescription for the necessary replacement cortisone.

He looked at it dully. 'Isn't that what you've been treating my wife with?'

'Yes,' I said, 'but you're having it for an entirely different reason. It should make you as well as it made her. Now, send your wife in, and I'll reduce her dosage.'

It had the desired effect on both of them. Within a few weeks, he looked a different man. When he came for one of his follow-up visits, I asked him if we had solved his other problem. He gave me a great beaming smile.

'Thank you, Doctor, yes it has,' but he did not elaborate.

When I got home that night, I could not help but notice how old and bedraggled both Emmy and Uncle Fred had become. Their unenthusiastic attempt at mating was not

167

successful.

'I wonder if I dare,' I thought to myself. 'What is the dose of cortisone for an elderly pair of geriatric geese, and how on earth could I administer it?'

15

One Sunday afternoon I was on the lawn, playing happily with a batch of young goslings, when my peace was rudely shattered as Rod came screaming up the drive in his old banger of a car.

Screaming was the right word. With loose gravel flying from behind his wheels, he accelerated viciously up to the house, the car skidding violently as he turned and braked hard.

The geese and I cowered in fear beneath a shower of small stones. When it stopped, as suddenly as it had begun, the little goslings rushed towards me and tried to hide underneath my trousers. Although none had been hurt, they were badly scared, and I was not feeling exactly civil myself.

Rod levered himself leisurely out of the car and slammed the door against the friction of its squealing hinges. He walked over to me, and the little birds milled about underneath me for protection. I dared not stand up, lest I squash one.

'You damned maniac!' I shouted up at him, as he ambled across the lawn. 'I've told you dozens of times that my drive isn't a race track.'

'Sorry, Doc,' he replied, not in the least contrite, and sat down beside me. 'I forgot.'

He drove everywhere like that, and when one old banger gave out under the strain, he acquired another. Out of a car, he never appeared to hurry, but his leisurely pace was deceptive.

Rod was a great believer in getting things done the easy way. He had got several things done for us already, some of them by quite worryingly dubious methods, waving aside questions about where he had obtained the materials.

Money never changed hands. Everything was by barter,

and the only thing that I had to barter was medical advice. In return I got sheds mended, fences erected and my heating and plumbing arrangements tidied up. Even the gravel with which he had just showered me so liberally, he had originally acquired for the drive.

On the few occasions when I had been asked to deal with some medical problem, it was never in the surgery, always at my home, and usually on a Sunday. He was not registered with us as a patient and would never have accepted a prescription. Whatever medication he needed had to be from a packet of samples in the back of my car, or something out of my bag.

I presumed that he needed something again today and looked at him enquiringly. He, however, was looking at the geese peeping out at him from under my trousers.

'Hell, boy,' he said, disbelief in his voice, 'they poor little sods think you're their mum.'

'That's right,' I said, 'they do.'

I picked one up and handed it to him. It wriggled out of his hand and scrabbled back to the safety of my legs. He watched in amazement. I rearranged the goslings beside me, so that none was in danger of being squashed, and waited for his request.

Whatever it was could wait. He was far too interested in the little geese which, having rapidly recovered from their fright, were trying to pick off the shiny metal buttons on his shirt sleeve. One, bolder than the others, jumped up on to his lap and began worrying the metal tag on his zip. It was soon joined by several more, investigating anything that was bright and metallic.

He played with them quite happily and was obviously in no hurry.

'You know,' he said after a while, 'there've been geese about at home for as long as I can remember, but our sods are as wild as hell. You can't get anywhere near them, and when we want one for the pot, I have to get the gun out and shoot it. Why are these so tame?'

'Well,' I explained, 'these little birds are extremely valuable, far too valuable to risk leaving with their parents. We give the parents some eggs of rubbishy old farmyard geese, and hatch these in the incubator. When they hatch out, they're a little lost and need a lot of looking after—they even have to be persuaded to eat.'

He nodded, and then hurriedly grabbed one that had just deposited a surprisingly large wet green mess on his shirt front.

'You little sod,' he said, as he wiped it off with a handful of grass. 'Sorry, Doc, you were saying?'

One more stain on his shirt, green or otherwise, would not be noticed among all the others. 'When they're first hatched,' I continued, 'they attach themselves to the first moving object that they see. Normally, this is mum, and it ensures that they stick with her all the time. Under our conditions, the first moving thing that they see is us. They fix on our voices, too. For the first day, we handle them as much as we can, talking to them the whole time, getting them to start eating. After the first twenty-four hours, they won't fix on anything, and if we don't get to them by then, they will be much wilder and more difficult to handle later, when they're half-grown.'

I pointed across to the old tennis court, where a slightly older batch were happily grazing. 'You see those there? They have to be taken back into the shed for warmth at night, but need to be out all day. Geese must have grass to eat. If they're reared in the shed all the time, the chicken food is much too rich for them. They eat far too much, grow far too quickly, and get problems with their legs. If they have grass all day and the other food all night, they grow well and stay healthy. Believe you me, catching them up and carting them about in a cardboard box twice a day is quite a chore. It's much easier to shout, "Come on, geese," and lead them in.'

At my shout, the batch in the tennis court all rushed to the gate and squeaked goosy greetings at me.

'You see,' I said. 'We shall have to go over and speak to them now, or they'll spend the rest of the afternoon running up and down the wire, trying to get out.'

Slowly we picked ourselves off the lawn and ambled over to the tennis court, followed by our little brood. After a few moments milling round our feet and cheeping indignantly at the younger goslings trying to hide beneath us, they returned quite happily to the serious business of eating grass.

'We'll just walk these little ones back to the shed,' I said to Rod, 'then we'll go and get that kettle on.' Rod always consumed gallons of tea, it was his staple diet.

While he drank, I waited for him to tell me why he had come, but he still seemed in no hurry and just wanted to know more about the geese. A good hour later, when I was beginning to believe that he had only come on a social call, he casually announced,

'It's my old Gran. She's got the belly ache. Wants to know if you could give her some jollop to settle it.'

'What sort of belly ache?' I asked.

'I dunno. Just belly ache.'

'Well, let's start at the beginning. How long's she had it?'

'Not really sure. About a week, I think. At least, that's how long she's been in bed.'

He paused, and helped himself to another mug of tea.

'It's not like old Gran to stay in bed for a week. Off her food, too. Been sick once or twice.'

He drank more tea.

'How bad's the pain?' I asked.

'Making her sweat a bit,' he said. 'Must be bad for her to ask me to get something for her. Never takes anything, normally.'

'How old is she?' I asked.

'Not sure, really. We reckon about ninety-two, but she could be a year or two more than that.' He shrugged his shoulders. 'Those pills you gave me when I had the squits, they sorted me out fairly smartish. Got any more of them?'

'No,' I said truthfully, not remembering just which batch of samples I had given him. 'You know, really, somebody ought to see her.' It did not sound the sort of occasion on which a lucky dip into the latest offerings of the drug companies was appropriate. I asked him who her normal doctor was.

'Normal doctor!' he repeated in some surprise. 'She hasn't seen a doctor in my lifetime. Nor my mother's, either, for that matter.'

'I'd better see her, then,' I said, making up my mind. 'Where does she live?'

'With me,' as if surprised that I did not know. I did not even know where Rod lived; all our dealings had been here.

'I'll get my car out,' I said, 'and follow you there.' I had no idea whether it would be a journey of five miles or fifty, and I certainly was not going to travel any distance in that old banger of his. It looked positively dangerous, if not lethal.

'OK,' he said, and we walked out of the kitchen.

My car was new and I was very proud of it. From his usual standing start, Rod left me miles behind. I did my best to keep up as we belted through the village, down the road to the river, and over the bridge into the marshes. After a couple of miles, without any warning, Rod performed one of his famous racing turns into a narrow gateway and, without changing speed, raced along the ever narrowing track beside the dyke. I just managed to stop and turn in after him, and proceeded at a much more civilised pace, jolting from bump to bump. My new car, I thought. This will wreck it.

By now, Rod was three fields away and out of sight. Gingerly, I followed his tracks through the mud and the potholes.

I must have followed that track along the dyke for at least another five miles before I caught him up. His car was parked in a sea of mud, with two rather miserable, half-starved cattle licking it. On the far side of the mud, a gaggle of nondescript, multicoloured geese cackled at me. Right in the centre was what can only be described as a small brick hovel, with a very low roof, and beside it some half-built brick walls and great heaps of roofing tiles, doors and window frames. They had obviously not been there very long. Rod was building himself a new house, and the materials were not arriving in progressive order.

'In here, Doc,' he called out, as he ducked under the very low roof and came out into the mud.

I squelched across to him and followed him in.

173

The old lady lay on a small low bed in the far corner, covered by a tangle of once brightly coloured and now very dirty blankets. The mud did not stop at the door, but continued inside. By half-way across the room it had dried somewhat, and whether the cottage had an earth floor or was merely exceedingly dirty, I should only be able to find out by digging into it with a spade. The only other furniture in the room was an equally dirty wooden table, and a couple of hard chairs.

I walked over to the old lady. 'Hello,' I said, and smiled at her. I did not know her name. Come to think of it, I did not know Rod's other name either, or even if he had one.

She looked back at me, half with hostility and half with relief. By the atmosphere, I was probably the first visitor inside the house for at least half a century.

'This is the Doc,' Rod said. 'I'll wait outside.' He ducked out of the door and was gone.

I looked for somewhere to sit. The bed was very low. It's a good job I'm wearing my goose-cleaning-out clothes, I thought to myself, as I pulled out one of the filthy chairs and placed it by her bedside.

'Dunno what he's sent for you for,' she grumbled. 'I'll be better in a day or two.'

'Well, now I've come, tell me all about it. I might be able to help.' I had already made a diagnosis. There was the characteristic smell of uraemia—kidney failure—in the air. But primary kidney failure was painless and insidious; her uraemia must be secondary to something else that was causing the pain.

I sat and waited for her to begin.

'It's just a belly ache,' she said, and repeated, 'I'll be better in a day or two.'

Gently, and with extreme reluctance on her part, I coaxed the story out of her. She had little more to add to Rod's version of events. A mild discomfort for several months, that had become progressively more severe until it had finally put her to bed and caused her to ask for help.

She was not accustomed to discussing her more intimate functions with complete strangers and had some difficulty in overcoming her natural inhibitions, but in spite of that,

174

her mind was crystal-clear, her memory unimpaired, and she was far from unintelligent.

'We'd better have a look at this tummy of yours,' I said, reaching out to pull down the blankets. She pulled them back up again, smartly.

'No man has laid a hand on my belly for the best part of seventy years,' she snapped, 'and I'm damned if one is going to start now.'

She glared at me, and I smiled back.

'Come off it,' I said. 'You know damned well neither of us is interested in that. If we want to do anything about this belly ache, we've got to know what's causing it.'

Her features relaxed a little, and she allowed me to pull down the scruffy blankets as far as her hips.

I could not believe it, not in this day and age, but there it was, right in front of my eyes. She was encased in several layers of underclothes that had been sewn on, all matted and glued together with a waxy grease. She was armour-plated from her knees to her elbows. I had always assumed that such customs had died out years ago.

I looked for an opening, or a join, to get at the skin. There was none.

'How do I, er, pull this up?' I murmured, fingering the soft, smooth, oily garment.

'You don't, you fool,' she snapped. 'Can't you see it's sewn on, and won't come off till it's cut off in the spring.'

Outside, it was a lovely warm May day, and I had goslings on the lawn at home. 'It's spring now,' I said.

'Not till June, it isn't,' she snapped again. 'That goose grease stays on till then.'

'For you, my dear,' I said, 'spring has come a little early this year. I'm going to cut if off now.'

I fetched the scissors from my bag and began to cut. She grumbled and swore, but allowed me to do it.

Underneath the goose grease, her skin was surprisingly clean and healthy. It was soft and almost unwrinkled, and looked much younger than the rest of her, that had been exposed to the air. Equally surprising was the size of her abdomen. It looked as if it contained a full-term pregnancy.

175

And on examination it did, too. A huge smooth mass rose out of her pelvis and reached almost up to her ribs. This was the cause of both her pain and the uraemia—an enormous ovarian cyst.

I replaced the flaps of greased cloth, and the dirty blankets.

'I'm going to die, aren't I?' she said in a matter-of-fact voice.

'No,' I replied. 'Not unless you want to.'

She pulled the blankets up under her chin. 'What, then?' she demanded.

'You've got this cyst,' I told her. 'It's pressing on your water-works, affecting your kidneys. You're being poisoned by your own waste products. The cyst has degenerated a bit, too; that's what's causing the pain.'

After a moment or two's silence, I added, 'It will have to come out, an operation. That will completely remove the pain and, with a bit of luck, your kidneys will start working again and you'll feel a new woman.'

She looked at me, giving the impression that she did not really believe a word I had said.

'And if I don't have the operation?'

'You'll die.'

'How long?'

'Hard to say. Depends on how long your kidneys last, but no more than two or three months. The pain will get worse, of course, but that won't kill you, and if I give you drugs for the pain, it'll be less.'

She considered it. 'Not got much option, have I, boy?'

'No,' I said. I stood up and replaced my things in my bag. 'I'll fix it all up with the hospital, and send an ambulance round for you later on this afternoon.'

'No. I'm having no ambulances here. Rod'll take me in.'

I ducked out under the door, and looked for him. I found him in some old sheds behind the skeleton of his new house, and explained the position to him.

'Give me time to get home and phone the hospital, won't you?'

'OK,' he nodded and, trying not to take too much of his mud into my car, I set off back up the track.

When I phoned the gynaecologist, he wouldn't believe me. 'Nobody sews themselves into goose grease,' he stated quite emphatically.

'Come and see for yourself,' I retorted. 'Then you can make the decision whether we operate tonight, or leave it till the list on Wednesday, after I've done all the blood tests.'

'Tonight,' he said. 'We'll do it tonight.'

The old lady was a model patient, despite the fact that the entire hospital staff were far more interested in her underwear than in her cyst. She answered all their questions with a refreshing bluntness. Before the operation, when the gynaecologist had finished examining her, she asked him flatly.

'Do you agree with him?'

He nodded, 'Yes,' and paused, looking thoughtful. 'But . . .'

'No buts,' she interrupted. 'Is it nasty? Is it cancer?'

'I don't think so, but we can't be sure till we've had a look inside.'

'If it's nasty, don't wake me up.' And she settled down to the business of being cut out of her winter warmth and prepared for the operation, quite sure that her last order would be obeyed.

The cyst was benign and weighed nine pounds when removed.

Two or three days after the operation, I found an enormous heap of new rolls of wire-netting piled up at the top of the yard.

'How did these get here?' I asked my wife, when I found them.

'Rod brought them,' she said. 'He asked me to tell you that his grandmother sent them.'

That night he brought a load of fencing posts, and by morning we had more than enough small runs to accommodate all the ever-increasing numbers of growing ducks and geese.

I tried to thank him, but he waved my words away. 'Didn't cost me nuthin', boy.'

'They didn't fall off the back of a lorry, did they?'

'Don't you worry about where they came from, boy. Somebody paid for 'em.'

Watching him drive off, showering gravel from behind his wildly spinning wheels, the nagging doubts I had entertained about being the inadvertent receiver of stolen property became a certainty. I walked slowly into the house, trying to make up my mind what to do about it. The 'phone was ringing.

'It's the old lady,' said the ward sister. 'She's collapsed.'

'I'm on my way,' I told her and, just as I was, in my gardening clothes, I set off for the hospital. This was most unexpected. The operation had been completely straightforward, and the old lady had that morning been taking her first tentative steps round the ward.

When I arrived, she was *in extremis*. She was blue, gasping for breath and complaining of severe pain in the chest. I gave her a large dose of heroin into a vein to ease the pain, and started to take a cardiograph. The first few squiggles on the paper showed that she had suffered a massive heart attack and, while I was still doing it, her old heart stopped. There was nothing that any of us could do.

The operation had been a great success, but the patient had died.

There was no way that we could contact Rod by 'phone, so I felt that I had better drive out and tell him. I was not exactly looking forward to being the bearer of such news, particularly as I had to confront him about the sources of the netting and posts.

I was driving slowly up his muddy track, pondering on how to combine the two tasks, when I saw that he had company. A builder's lorry, laden with bricks, was being unloaded. Rod looked very embarrassed and discomforted as I squelched through the mud towards him. Waving him to one side, out of earshot of the two men unloading the lorry. I told him about his grandmother. 'I'm sorry,' I added lamely. 'We did everything that we could.'

He was absolutely shattered. It had never even crossed his mind that she might die. They were genuine tears he shed, but they were interrupted by a shout from one of the men unloading the bricks.

'Hey, look! It's the bloody police!'

We both looked up the track. Three police cars were coming down it, fast.

The two men unloading the lorry started to run. 'Stupid sods,' grunted Rod, as he wiped his streaming eyes with his fist. 'They won't get far. They can be seen for miles.'

Feeling that my presence was now an embarrassment not only to Rod, but to myself as well, I walked back to the car, trying hard not to collect too much mud on the way.

I met the police cars several fields away. They stopped me, and I became only too conscious of all that wire-netting festooned so conspicuously about my property, as a policeman leaped out of one of the cars and walked briskly over to me. It was Steve, one of the officers from the town.

He recognised me as he came nearer and, leaning on the car window, said jokingly, 'New car, eh, Doc? Not stolen property from up there, is it?'

Covered in guilt and blushing profusely. I shook my head negatively.

'Well, what are you doing here then?' and, carrying his joke far too near for comfort, 'Come to buy some stolen bricks?'

With as much dignity as I could muster, I said, 'No. His old grandmother collapsed and died this afternoon. I had just come out to let him know.'

Steve looked a bit crestfallen. 'Sorry, Doc. I didn't know.'

'He's taken it very badly,' I added. 'He's more than a bit upset.'

'Not half as upset as he's going to be when we get there.' All sympathy had gone from his face. 'We've caught him red-handed with that lorry there. We reckon he's moved thousands of pounds' worth of stuff in the last year or so. We've got him this time.'

All that wire-netting. I tried to speak, but no sound came.

'Best be on your way,' said Steve. 'If you hang about here, you might get involved. I'll see you later.'

An abject, guilt-ridden coward, I drove off.

179

Much later that night, Steve called at the house. I invited him in and offered him a drink.

'Thanks,' he said, 'I'll have a scotch. I'm technically off duty.'

I poured myself a very large one, and worried how I could bring up the subject of the wire-netting before he did.

'Won't be seeing Rod about for the next year or two,' he said casually, as he lowered himself comfortably into a chair and sipped his drink.

I took a large swig of mine.

'Got him properly this time. He's confessed to about twenty more.'

He looked so comfortable and relaxed.

'That wire-netting. Up my yard. That was stolen too, was it?'

'No,' he said, unconcernedly sipping my whisky. 'That was one of the things we checked on. He paid for that, and,' he added, smiling broadly, 'he paid for the gravel in your drive, too.'

I stared at him, dumbfounded.

'Rod,' I said to the world in general, 'I owe you an apology.' I raised my glass. 'Your very good health. I'll see you when you come out.'

Steve drank. 'To when he comes out.' I recharged both our glasses. 'Tell me,' he said, 'is it true that the old lady was covered in goose grease, and sewn up all winter in her underclothes?'

16

At some stage in its life, the house had been owned by a complete philistine. The people from whom we bought it had only owned it for a few years, and for most of those years had been mainly abroad. They had kept their home base beautifully clean and aired and maintained, but had done nothing in the way of improvements or alterations.

The decorations, too, were unaltered from the days of the philistine. It was difficult, if not impossible, to work out who the philistine had been, from the long list of owners and mortgagees, so carefully documented in the deeds.

The poor old house had changed hands so many times, that even the ghosts in the attic must have become confused.

We gathered, from various sources, that the earliest mention of habitation on the site was in the seventh century, when some devout and earnest monk had tried to convert the heathen living in the area, and had recorded the narrowness of his escape from death in the Anglo-Saxon Chronicle.

The next historical mention of it was in 1342, when the Manorial Rolls for that year recorded that the absentee landlord had been fined twelve shillings and sixpence for failing to hold the annual Moot Court.

Just after the time of the Spanish Armada, it had come into the hands of some splendid old pirate, whose family had held it until the time of the First World War, when the whole estate had been broken up and sold off in little pieces.

We also gathered, from the same sources, that in 1660 the original house had been completely demolished and rebuilt, and then again, in 1895, it had been totally altered and modernised to the taste of that period.

The deeds, unfortunately, were not a great source of

ancient information; they only went back to the great sale of 1916. Apparently the old parchments, with the Great Seal of Queen Elizabeth the First, William Pitt the Elder, Charles James Fox, and many others, were all stored in an old oak charter chest. This chest originally came from one of the galleons of the Spanish Armada and had been stolen, complete with all the deeds, in the chaos of the sale. Our information was village hearsay only.

Virtually everybody who had owned it since the great dispersal sale had added his little bit of history to it.

Two enormous egg-washing rooms, and an even bigger games room above them, had been added to the back by the gentleman who tried to cash in on the egg boom. He had failed and been obliged to sell the place, but his egg-washing rooms remained.

A swimming pool had been dug in the west-facing terrace, presumably by the philistine, for he had omitted to put any filtration arrangements in it, and had sited it under an enormous plane tree, whereupon it promptly filled with rotting leaves. His successor had put a greenhouse type of structure over the top of the lot, to keep out the leaves. This was most successful, for they all lay on the roof, getting thicker year by year. Inside this edifice, the setting sun did manage to penetrate sufficiently to evaporate a little water and condense it on the glass. Green algae found this continual dampness a perfect habitat, and dripped with the water on the glass back into the swimming pool, turning that deep green also, despite gallons of chlorine and other chemicals. The temperature of the water remained a steady fifty-five degrees fahrenheit, summer and winter—the perfect temperature for storing either wine or cheese, but not to swim in. The surveyor's report before we bought the house gave a high probability of the lot collapsing in the very near future, but so far it had held up.

Inside the house, the ravages of the philistine, or his friends and successors, remained. The main sitting-room, virtually thirty-five feet square and of beautiful proportions, had originally been panelled in oak throughout. Village gossip recorded that one impecunious owner, in a desperate attempt to salvage his fortunes, had stripped it out and sold it. All the old oak doors had gone as well, and been replaced by cheap home-made efforts of hollow hardboard and glass panels. Even that had not saved him, for he had sold the place soon after his desecration of it.

Insult had been added to the injury already inflicted on that room. The old fireplace had been removed at the same time as the panelling, and replaced with a modern monstrosity. This was an incredible structure of polished plastic stone, stretching right across the room in a series of shelves and alcoves. Every few feet, cheap and nasty wrought-iron imitations of various sizes of cartwheel had been nailed into it, so that they revolved, groaning hideously as they did so.

The whole was not resting securely on the floor, where it should have been, but six inches above it, and the resulting space was filled with a board, into which lighted bottle ends had been inserted. There was, mercifully, no apparent way in which the light bulbs in the bottles could be changed without dismantling the whole structure, and over the years the lot had died of shame.

Another philistine, or perhaps the same one, had tried growing mushrooms in the ancient cellars. He had carted in several tons of a mixture of horse manure, peat and chalk, which was still there. The mushroom growing had been a complete disaster, for a much stronger strain of ancient fungi, one of the many species of dry rot, had taken over the culture medium from the weaker mushroom, and flourished mightily.

This must all have been done before the philistine had cemented up the outer door to the cellar, as part of the construction of his swimming pool. The only way out now for all that fungating muck was in forkfuls up the narrow stairs, to a wheelbarrow in the hall. However, it had now lain there undisturbed for so long that moving it out came very low on my list of priorities. If it was going to grow into the fabric of the building, it had already done so, and we had no immediate plans to open up the cellars and improve the pop music scene.

Heading my list of priorities was the decoration in the

dining-room. This again was a beautifully proportioned room, some thirty feet by twenty, with a very high ceiling. It was obviously much older than many other parts of the house, for the ceiling was supported by a venerable hand-hewn oak beam, running the length of the room.

The fireplace, too, was the original walk-in size, occupying virtually the whole of one wall, but with the old wooden beams replaced by crisp, modern white-painted wood, squared and symmetrical. The old bricks lining the fireplace had been painted bright yellow, and the mortar, pillar-box red. Stuck on to this red and yellow horror at the back was a small council-house-type firegrate, surrounded by garish lilac-blue tiles, stuck on by a one-eyed amateur who was looking the other way when he did it.

The overall effect was quite repulsive, especially when all attempts to light a fire failed, with only a smoke-filled room to show for the effort.

The vandalised effect of the fireplace was not out of keeping with the rest of the room. The one long outer wall had been virtually replaced with an enormous plate-glass window, more appropriate to a high street shop than an old manor house, and this looked out into the green gloom of the swimming pool room. The opposite wall was papered with bamboo stalks, three feet apart, and apparently growing from floor to ceiling. I could not sit at the table facing them; the sense of vertigo induced by subconsciously trying to find a focal point in their endless vertical structure quite put me off my food.

Just to complete the disturbing atmosphere created by the rest of the room, the ceiling above that glorious old beam had been painted black, and covered with thousands of bright little aluminium stars.

However, we could live with it, as we had done for these first years. A soon as we had earned some money, we told ourselves frequently, we would make a start. Naturally, in my ignorance, I assumed that we would start on the dining-room.

*   *   *

Anyone who has owned, or lived in, an old house, knows from bitter experience that the fundamentals must always come first. In our case, these were the kitchen sink and the electric wiring. Both had appeared to be in good heart when we moved in, and both within a short while were defunct.

The kitchen sink was the first to go. Nothing dramatic: it just took longer and longer to empty. A half-inch of greasy, cold water lying permanently in the bottom of it became the norm.

A gas-gun was acquired, one that was widely advertised as capable of clearing anything. According to the advertisement, all one had to do was insert the business end into the plug hole, charge it with a small cylinder of carbon dioxide, and pull the trigger.

What should have happened, according to the advertisement, was the rapid and permanent movement of the obstruction, shot as if from a rifle barrel, down the pipe and away.

What actually happened was totally different and utterly unexpected. In the advertisement, a very pretty young lady in a white coat floated from blocked sink to blocked sink, confounding armies of hairy spanner-laden plumbers on the way. I did not have the army of plumbers watching, just the family, all crowding in to get a better view. All of them had seen the advertisement and naturally were expecting the presumed miraculous result.

The sink was brimful of dirty water. I charged the gun, rolled up my sleeves and inserted the nozzle into the plug hole, placing my finger firmly on the trigger according to instructions. The children chanted the countdown: 'Five, four, three, two, one. PULL!'

I pulled. The resulting explosion covered everything within a radius of ten feet in greasy washing-up water. The children leaped about in pain and delight as they tried to get the soapy water out of their eyes, and somebody's wife went into one of her famous chilly silences as she quietened the children from within the ruins of her new dress, and mopped up the mess.

Order restored, I tried again. This time the audience

stood well back and the whole sink was draped in wet towels. It was a very satisfactory, controlled explosion. I got a shirtful of water, but something seemed to have happened down that plug hole, for the sink began slowly to empty.

With great satisfaction, I watched the greasy water flow away.

Imperceptibly at first, and then with growing alarm, I began to feel that all was not well. My feet were getting wet.

Close inspection revealed that all I had done was to blow the fittings off the bottom of the sink. Buckets and mops were summoned, while the chilly silence grew chillier.

We now had a very big problem, for I had not realised before I started that the sink had been installed by the philistine. It stood, as part of a table and work bench, as an island unit in the middle of the room. His knowledge of plumbing had been rudimentary, and his ruler must have been made of elastic, for where the various bits and pieces should have joined, in a nice water-tight fit, they did not. He had crudely cut off the non-aligned joints and cobbled the lot together with glue. My controlled explosion had blown it all apart, never to be rejoined.

Worse was to come. The outlet pipe was still blocked and, on a closer look, the reason was obvious. Instead of using proper plumbing fittings to make the various bends needed in the one-inch copper pipe, the philistine had used one long length and merely bent it across his knee to get it to fit. At each of these bends the pipe had flattened, so that the whole system was virtually blocked before it had ever been used.

In horror, I traced the pipe to the floor. This mangled, malformed travesty of a modern plumbing system had been concreted in, beneath the kitchen floor. To restore the central purpose of our kitchen I had got to dig it up.

But the sink functioned, so long as a bucket was strategically placed beneath it, and a relay of willing legs humped the waste water to an outside drain at increasingly frequent intervals.

It was quite remarkable how, whenever it looked as if

work was in the offing, an audience of small boys rapidly disappeared. Humping buckets was work, to be avoided at all costs. As if by magic, they all disappeared. Only the chilly silence of their mother remained, and that did not last long.

We sat on the wet floor and giggled. It was just too much.

Major repairs of this nature were beyond my simple skills. While still sitting in my puddle on the floor, wondering what to do about it, the 'phone rang. Another of those calls from the hospital.

'I know you're not on duty, but can you come at once?'

I went. At least I did have sufficient simple skills to deliver a distressed baby, even though my mind was on my plumbing as I did it. It did not take long to rotate him to the correct position, apply the forceps and then bring him gently into the world, but it took nearly an hour to revive him. The poor little mite was badly shocked when I drew him out, but yelling his head off nicely when I left.

Back home, three little faces met me at the back door. 'The Benny man's come to mend the sink you blew up,' they announced. I had not noticed his car in the yard.

He was on his knees, with his head in the cupboard under the sink, and a stream of extremely coarse language conveyed his opinion of the ignorant idiots who had installed the system, and of those who had blown it up.

'Evening, Benny,' I said to his upturned backside.

'Evenin', Doc,' he replied, pausing briefly in his blasphemous monologue, but he did not come out of the cupboard.

I looked at Ruth. 'He just turned up,' she said. 'He must be psychic.'

'Perhaps the ghosts told him,' I whispered in her ear, but she shushed me as Benny ponderously reversed out from under the sink.

'Whole lot's had it,' he pronounced. 'We'll need a complete new sink and fittings, and a new discharge pipe.'

All I could do was agree.

We sat at the table and drank coffee. 'Damn' silly place to put a sink in the first place, in the middle of a room,' he

187

said after a while. 'It'll cost a lot less, and be a lot easier to do, if we put it back under the window where it belongs.'

Once more, all I could do was agree.

'I'll be over tomorrow night. We can knock this lot out,' waving at the sink unit and attached table, 'and I'll order the new one for the night after.'

Passing his cup to Ruth for more coffee, he said to her, 'Go and choose one from Tatler's, and tell them it's for me. My cousin Harry's on the desk. He'll give it you, trade.'

He came as arranged the next night, and we spent most of the evening looking for stop-cocks to turn the water off. In the end he did it by flattening the pipes with a hammer. It took but a moment to remove the taps and sinktop and, flexing his muscles, he set about the brickwork of the sink unit. His sledgehammer flew through the air with venom. After about ten minutes he had slightly cracked one brick.

'What the hell?' he muttered to himself, as he put down the hammer and began to inspect the barely damaged brick. 'Come and look at this, Doc,' he said. 'The last time I saw this stuff was when we used it to make the vaults at Barclay's Bank. It's the same cement they use for building prisons. Look at this,' and he stared at it in amazement. 'The stupid sod's even put the reinforcing metal bars in!'

For the remainder of that night, we took it in turns to wield the sledgehammer. All we had to show for our efforts were three powdered bricks. The rest remained untouched.

'Can't think where he got this stuff from,' Benny said, 'unless it fell off the back of a lorry and he got it cheap. We can only hope the bloke who sold it to him's behind bars, held up by the same stuff.'

For several nights we laboured at moving it, interrupted on my part by being on call.

Ruth, as instructed, went down to Tatler's builders' merchants to choose her sink, and came back bubbling. She had seen not only the sink she wanted, but also the entire kitchen, the whole displayed in their show-room.

'Was it expensive?' I deigned to ask.

'Very,' she nodded, 'but it was the kitchen I've always dreamed about having,' and seeing the look on my face, 'but I only ordered the sink.'

Thankfully, I resumed my shift on the sledgehammer. Out of the corner of my eye, I could see her listening intently to Benny, looking very conspiratorial. Glancing up, I caught his eye.

'Leave this to me, Doc,' he said.

*   *   *

When I arrived home the next evening, late, tired and hungry, the new kitchen furniture was piled high in the centre of the room. I stared at it aghast.

'S'all right, Doc,' Benny grinned at me. 'Got you a good bargain. Cousin Harry told me they always sell off their display units cheap to the trade. We had to take the lot, though, thirty per cent list price.'

I stared at it again. 'Thirty per cent of what?' I asked.

'Now that would be telling,' he grinned. 'Never asked him.'

We now had not only a new sink, but two cookers, two fridges, two eye-level grills, and God knew what else besides. There seemed, to my tired and inexperienced eyes, to be enough units and cupboards to go round the room twice.

Benny pointed to a large cardboard box sitting on the floor, all sealed up with sticky tape, with an envelope neatly taped to the top. 'Old Man Tatler brought it out himself,' he remarked. 'Said I was to give it to you personally.' He dismissed it with a derogatory wave of his hand. 'He's a mean old sod, it's only the bill, and the screws and fittings.'

My supper appeared and was served on the top of one of the units.

'Come and eat this first,' Ruth said, 'before you open that bill. Envelopes with bills in should never be opened on a empty stomach.'

'No,' I said, 'let's get it over with first. Bad news after food always gives me indigestion,' and, taking my penknife out of my pocket, I slashed the tape and pulled off the envelope. In doing so, I lifted one flap open on the top of

189

the box. The tops of a row of bottles looked back at me.

'These aren't screws and fittings,' I said as I took one out. It was a very expensive-looking bottle of wine.

We stared at each other, and the bottle, in amazement. 'Open the envelope,' Ruth said softly. I ripped it open. It was a bill from Tatler's, only instead of typed columns of figures, an elderly, unsteady hand had scrawled across it, 'With many grateful thanks for my grandson, and with the compliments of Charles Tatler.'

I passed the piece of paper to Ruth and, after reading it, she passed it silently to Benny.

'Well I'll be damned,' he said quietly, passing it back. 'I didn't know the mean old sod had it in him.'

'Your supper's getting cold,' Ruth remarked as we stared dumbfounded at each other.

I sat down at the makeshift table, placing the bottle of wine beside my plate. It was a very expensive bottle of wine, but the more I thought about it, the more appropriate it seemed to drink it now. I caught Ruth's eye and she read my thoughts. Silently she produced three glasses and a corkscrew. I opened the bottle and solemnly poured us each a glass.

'To the Tatler grandson,' I said, 'whoever he may be, because I don't think I've met him.'

Open-mouthed, both Benny and Ruth stared at me, their glasses half-way up.

'Could it have been the baby you delivered on Tuesday—you know, the night you blew up the sink?' asked Ruth.

'I don't know,' I replied. 'I didn't ask the woman's name. I've done several in the last few weeks. The name Tatler doesn't ring a bell, and I'm sure they're not patients of mine. If it was a baby I've delivered, he could be any one of several.'

'It was the one on Tuesday,' Benny interrupted. 'Cousin Harry did mention it. Didn't you know, didn't you recognise her?'

'No,' I had to admit. 'It was all rather panic situation. It was obvious that I had to get him out fast, and then I was too busy trying to revive him. Once he'd come round, I just

190

said goodnight and left. She was just another emergency forceps delivery that I had to do, because no one else could have got there in time.'

'She thinks the world of you,' Benny said in disbelief. 'Young Tom Tatler's singing your praises all over town, says you were a perfect gentleman.' And with the disbelief still all over his face, 'And you didn't know who she was?'

'No,' I repeated. 'It never crossed my mind to ask her name, and it wouldn't have made any difference if I had.'

I began to eat. 'Your health, young Tatler,' I said as I graced my supper with his grandfather's wine.

As I ate, Benny started digging holes in the floor with a pickaxe. Mercifully the wine mellowed his language, as he discovered that the philistine had brought in the cold water pipe from one side of the room, and the hot from the other, and concreted the lot in with more of the bank vault cement. In the end, he had to dig up most of the floor to take the water to the new sink under the window. It would have been a lot less trouble, and infinitely less expensive, just to have replaced the offending waste pipe and left the sink where it was.

Eventually, however, the job was done and the new sink installed and functional, together with the waste disposal unit and dishwashing machine that we found among the job lot of kitchen units.

It took nearly three more weeks of solid evening work to arrange and instal the remainder of the kitchen units. Plans were drawn up and redrawn several times. All the old cupboards and other fittings had to be removed, but eventually we had everything placed in its final position. As might have been expected, there were more problems. All these beautiful new units were geometrically square, and fitted together in a nice straight line. The walls and the corners of our old house did not.

Another cousin of Benny's, this one called Len, a plasterer by trade, had to be summoned, to completely replaster the walls and render them fit to receive our new equipment. He also retiled the floor.

When, it seemed like months later, the job was finally completed and we had all gathered to open another bottle

191

of Old Man Tatler's wine, I felt content with my lot. My wife was in seventh heaven in her new kitchen, and Benny's charges for his labours had not been excessive.

Little did I realise how short-lived it would all be. I was blissfully unaware of the rotting electric wiring smouldering around us, of the fact that Old Tatler's generosity extended only as far as the wine and did not include his kitchen units, of the fact that the monstrous fireplace raised six inches off the floor was only supported by planks of wood already half burned through and, worst of all, that I should have to live with those vertiginous bamboo stalks for another three years. Had I know, too, that the fungus-bearing mushroom manure in the cellar was a time bomb, already primed to go off, I should probably have sold up and emigrated.

I did not know. I was happy and enjoyed the wine.

17

'I'm afraid he's gone, Mrs Long,' I shouted at her, and moved to pull the sheets up over his face.

She was partly in my way and, as I went to step round her, she put a hand on my arm to stop me, at the same time screwing up the volume control of her hearing aid with the other. It emitted a howling screech, inaudible to her but mind-paralysing to me.

'I can see you're saying something,' she said, 'but Lord only knows what it was.'

As so often when I wanted to communicate with her, I waved both hands across my chest in the traditional 'no good' manner, then took the screeching hearing aid out of her ear, traced the long cord to somewhere inside her commodious apron and removed the battery box. With relief, I turned it off.

'Oh dear,' she said, 'was it annoying you again?'

I nodded my head. 'Yes.'

She stood looking at me with her head on one side, like a small sparrow; only she was not a small sparrow, she was fifteen stone of tough old lady, and I had to tell her in a combination of sign language and lip reading that her husband had just died.

It should not be too difficult, I thought, for we had both been expecting it for over a year and, after all, he was eighty-six. Poor old Cecil Long had suffered a massive stroke which had left him completely paralysed all down his left side, incontinent and helpless. His mind, however, had been completely unaffected.

Resenting bitterly his crippled condition, especially the catheter and disposable nappies that he had been forced to wear, he had not been a model patient. He had refused on principle to take any medication whatsoever, on the grounds that he would be better off dead and had no wish to prolong his intolerable life; and he accepted with very bad grace the devoted attentions of is wife and the district nurse.

The only people to whom he could express his venom were these two good ladies, and at times his ungrateful remarks were vindictive and spiteful. Every day the contractures of his useless limbs had to be forced straight and his joints exercised, to prevent his limbs going into spasm. If spasm did occur the pain was excruciating, for although the stroke had destroyed that part of his brain that controlled the movement of his left side, it had left his appreciation of pain completely unaffected.

He had not been easy to live with before his stroke, and afterwards had been impossible. Now, mercifully, he had died at last, going peacefully in his sleep. There had been so many false alarms, and the longer that it went on, the greater the shock when it finally happened.

I looked her full in the face and shook my head sadly, and she concentrated on my lips. There was no point in shouting, as without her hearing aid she could hear nothing. I mouthed the words: 'I'm afraid he's gone.'

She nodded. 'I thought he had. Poor old thing, he hated living like that, you know.'

'I'd better tell the nurse,' I started to say, but realised that there would be no need as I heard the distinctive sound of her car coming up the drive. Nurse Scrivens, although magnificent at her job, had no mechanical sense whatever. She firmly believed that putting the car into top gear might strain it, so only used that gear in cases of dire necessity. Most of the time she drove, with the engine screaming, in bottom gear. The exhaust system was distinctly deficient in several vital parts, but it never bothered her, as she could not hear it above the noise of the engine.

She bustled into the room, sized up the situation in two seconds flat and, as was her wont, took complete charge of everything. She put her great beefy arms round Mrs Long in a motherly embrace and hugged her close for a few moments; then with sufficient volume to make me jump a foot in the air, bellowed down her ear, 'Go and make some tea. I'll see to him.'

Mrs Long moved meekly off into the kitchen, silent tears

194

welling out of her eyes. Nurse Scrivens brushed her apron straight with her hands, its crisp starch rustling, with each unnecessary stroke driving her own emotions behind its smooth front. In their different ways, they had both been very fond of the irascible old man.

With her own stiff upper lip firmly in place, she said, 'I always like to see them cry at this stage; makes it easier later on.' She set about laying out poor old Cecil. 'Go and ring the undertakers,' she commanded, 'and tell them to come and take him to the chapel of rest.'

Like Mrs Long, I went off meekly to do as I was told.

In the eyes of the law, the body could not be moved until I had either issued a death certificate or authorised the removal myself, prior to issuing one.

There was no point in reminding Nurse Scrivens of this; in most cases, like this one, it was only a formality. I 'phoned the undertakers and joined Mrs Long in the kitchen. She had made the tea and, out of habit, poured four cups. I said nothing, and sat at the table beside her. The tears were streaming openly down her face now, and I held her hand to give her what comfort I could.

She would miss him terribly, I thought. They had been married for more than sixty years, but there were no children and they had kept themselves very much to themselves for at least the last twenty years. Since his stroke, she had devotedly nursed him and waited on his every need, and it had been a full-time job. The empty days stretched uninvitingly ahead.

Her only company would be her cats. There must have been nearly a dozen of them, long-legged, mainly white creatures, with patches of various colours scattered irregularly over their coats, and evil-looking oriental eyes that stared back at you. Mrs Long did not seem overfond of them. She fed them daily, but they lived mainly in the garden, reproducing prolifically to keep up their numbers, while the estate keeper did his best to keep them down when they invaded his pheasant pens each spring.

The children loved to come with me to see Mrs Long and her pussy cats. What the fascination was, I did not know, for we had plenty of cats at home, but they played happily in the garden with them while I went in to see poor old Cecil. Perhaps it was because they had a job to catch one to play with, and it was more of a cat hunt, or perhaps it was because of the special jam scones Mrs Long fed them with afterwards.

Seeing her fuss round the children, and the totally natural empathy that so quickly developed between them, it always seemed to me sad that she had never had any family of her own to fuss over, only the cantankerous old Cecil.

We drank our tea and I took my leave of them. Even though I had the death certificate book in the car, I said that I would bring it out the next day, purely as an excuse to call and see her. I knew the nurse would do the same, with a similar excuse.

One or both of us called every day for the next week or so, and drank the inevitable cup of tea, but she seemed to be coping well with her lonely life. Neither the nurse nor I was able to go to the funeral. I wished that I had made the effort when I read an account of it in the local paper: she and the vicar were the only people present. Alone they had lived, self-sufficient, and alone she had buried him. In the solitude of her total silence, she would be more alone than ever, and only her cats for company.

Over the following weeks, I called sporadically to see her, when passing that way, and asked the social services to take her under their wing. They offered her a place in several old folk's homes, but all offers were politely refused. Her landlord, who badly needed the house for his newly appointed farm foreman, had his offer of alternative accommodation equally politely declined. 'This is my home,' she told them all. 'I've lived here nearly all my life and I intend to die here.' And that was the end of the conversation.

In the end, the landlord did manage to persuade her to live in only half of the rambling old farmhouse, and he divided it into two, leaving her their old kitchen and sitting-room downstairs, and her bedroom, one other room and the bathroom upstairs. This seemed to me to be a very fair arrangement, for not only did it reduce her rent considerably, it also gave her company in the form of her new neighbours.

During the alterations, she was under the feet of the workmen all day, and they drank gallons of her tea. There being no real need for me to visit her regularly, and with other things on my mind, I stopped calling frequently, and the frequently dropped down to occasionally, and then stopped.

*   *   *

The months passed. Not having to think about Mrs Long, I had almost forgotten her existence in the press of other people's problems.

I was forcibly reminded that she did exist when Peter, the village policeman, phoned me up late one evening. To be more precise, it was nearly midnight.

'It's about Mrs Long,' he said. 'You haven't by any chance put her into hospital today?'

'No,' I replied. 'I haven't seen the old lady for weeks. What's the problem?'

'She's disappeared,' he said, 'and we've got a spot of bother here that she could be the cause of, but I thought that I had better check with you that it is Mrs Long. I could have looked a fool if you had put her into hospital today.'

I repeated my denial and asked him to tell me all about it. I could see him in my mind consulting his notebook as he did so.

'Number one,' he said. 'We've had a phone call from her every night for the past week, telling us to come at once, there are burglars in her attic.'

He paused to clear his throat. 'But she didn't ring to-night, and I thought that we'd cured her. The first time that she called, I went myself and took it seriously, but there was nobody there. I even looked in the loft. When she rang again the next night, I went round and gave her a good ticking off and, after that, whenever she rang I asked one of the boys in the patrol panda to drop in and put her back to bed. The trouble is, the new sergeant from Leapton was on last night, and he turned up with three squad cars and the dog van.'

I could visualise him smiling, for the amusement was coming through in his voice.

'Her cats set about the dog, and there was one hell of a fight all over the house. The dog's badly scratched about the face, one of the cats was killed, and the dog handler has put in an official complaint. Worst of the lot, the sergeant was bitten through the hand trying to separate them.'

'And I suppose you're on the carpet for not officially reporting all her previous calls?' I asked.

He did not answer my question directly, merely hesitated and then continued. 'Number two. She's accused her neighbour of stealing all her garden tools.'

I remembered that, on one of my visits some months back, she had said the same to me, but I had dismissed it then as being nonsense. She had not done any gardening for several years, and the new farm foreman had taken over the whole garden and ploughed it, leaving her just a small patch of lawn to hang her washing out. He had even kept that mown for her.

At the time, I had spoken to him about it and we had both treated it as a joke. What tools remained were pathetic remnants of a bygone age, with rotten and worm-eaten handles. He had been quite upset by the accusation, as he had gone to a lot of trouble to befriend and help the old lady.

I told Peter all about it.

'I know,' he said, 'but she's written to the Chief Constable about it, complaining that I'm neglecting my duties, and I've got to give him a full report.'

Knowing just how much he detested paperwork, I sympathised.

'Number three,' he went on. 'Ben Baker, her landlord, has been in this morning. She's refused to pay any rent since her husband died, and he's brought me a whole sheaf of abusive letters, accusing him of just about everything from rape to bigamy. He says he'll take her to court if I don't stop her writing them.'

The letters must have been very nasty, for Ben was one

of the old-style feudal landlords, whose family had owned the estate for several generations. Cecil had originally worked for his grandfather and, after his retirement, had continued to live in the old farmhouse. Ben had a very strong feeling of obligation to the old family retainers; the non-payment of the rent, a fraction of what he could have got, would have worried him not at all. The letters obviously had, as they probably referred to some misdemeanours of his youth that he thought were forgotten.

'Number four, and this is the real reason I'm ringing you at this time of night, is that she's out somewhere in the village in her nightdress, and I don't know if you've noticed, but it's raining like hell. I've got all the search parties out, and when we find her you'll have to get her in somewhere. We can't just take her home and leave her.'

I agreed that I should certainly have to see her and do something when they found her. 'How do you know she's out in her nightdress?' I asked him.

He chuckled. 'You know young Billy Wright, the tearaway who fancies himself with the ladies?' I did indeed know young Billy Wright. Ever since he had had the mumps a few years ago, he was convinced that he was sterile and that sex was purely for pleasure, not only for him, but also for as many young girls as he could persuade to enjoy it with him. He had had tremendous success convincing them that he was harmless, and as he seemed to be rather good at it, quite a few had had a go with him, purely for the fun of it, they told me afterwards. Billy himself was quite convinced that, being sterile, his powers would soon leave him, and he had better get in as much as possible while he was able.

Unfortunately for the girls, he was far from sterile, and there was an epidemic of unwanted pregnancies in the village, and a posse of irate fathers and frustrated boyfriends threatening to remove his powers for good with a veterinary instrument if they ever caught him.

Billy had wisely got a job in the town and now did his courting there. His powers and persuasion were undiminished, but at least he now had an arrangment with the local chemist to get his contraceptives wholesale.

199

'Well,' he continued, 'young Billy was apparently on the job with a girl—she's only here on holiday for a week—and they were hard at it in Hangman's Wood when this ghost, an old lady with tangled grey hair and a billowing white dress, rushed up at them moaning and shrieking.'

He chuckled again. 'Confucius was right, you know. Girl with skirt up runs faster than boy with trousers down. Rape impossible. She was twenty yards ahead when they passed my house, and they were both going like hell.'

Still chuckling, he went on, 'I saw them from the window, and thought I'd better see what was going on. I'd just got into the road, when this car comes up, and the driver tells me that he nearly ran down an old woman in a white nightdress running down the road. I've got Billy and the girl here now, both too scared to go home. Might teach him a lesson, but there's no sign of Mrs Long. I've been up to her house—the door's wide open, and no sign of her.'

I agreed I had better come out and help with the search party.

When I arrived, Billy and his girl were still there, white and shaking, and clutching mugs of hot coffee liberally laced with rum—I could smell it from the door. The new sergeant from Leapton was also there, his arm in a sling and white bandages right down to his fingers. Although he never actually said it, his whole attitude expressed the feeling that he hoped both Mrs Long and her cats would depart peacefully of exposure during the night.

We waited impatiently for news. There was none. The various search parties came and went, with nothing to report. Billy and the girl began to look a little less pale and scared, but neither of them dared go outside into the dark. I presumed that the police would take them home later.

The hours passed very slowly; my watch said it was two a.m. I knew that the minute I went home to bed, the 'phone would ring to say that they had found her and I would only have to come out again, so I stayed. The longer I stayed, the more likely it became that they would find her any minute, and the more loth I was to go. I had just made up my mind that it would be sensible to get some sleep, if only a little, when the 'phone rang.

200

We all jumped expectantly to attention as the sergeant answered it. No, they had not found Mrs Long, but the girl's father had reported her missing and was on his way to claim her.

Billy's face went deathly white. It was not his night; although no one had asked her age, she was probably under sixteen. Even though the father would be unaware of his record, and would not come armed with the necessary veterinary instrument, I could see that young Billy was in for a very hot and painful session. It seemed a suitable moment to go.

Wearily I climbed into my car, and the sergeant said he would call me out if they needed me.

It had stopped raining, the wind had dropped completely and the temperature had gone down several degrees. A white mist was forming over the fields, rolling down from the slightly higher ground into the hollows. It was quite eerie, and definitely not the night to be out in nothing but a soaking wet nightdress, lost in the fog. I hoped they found the poor old thing soon.

The road home was slightly undulating. On the crests the fog only came up to the car's headlights, so that they shone above it, and as the road dipped, visibility suddenly became virtually nil, as every particle of fog reflected the light in a great white blanket.

Concentrating totally on my driving, I emerged from a slight hollow and, as the lights momentarily lifted out of the ground mist and then dropped back into it, I saw an apparition. One moment it was there, and then it had vanished: a white face, with a fringe of grey hair, mouth wide open as if screaming, and arms raised up in supplication.

Instinctively, as I saw it in front of the car, I had jammed on the brakes in an emergency stop, with sufficient force to stall the engine. I sat there, in the total silence, shaking from head to foot, staring out through the windscreen at the will-o-the-wisp mist as it rose and fell in front of me, and little fingers of it billowed and eddied like waves on the sea.

There was nothing there, only me and the mist, and total

201

silence.

I remained there, stupefied with shock and quite unable to act or think, for what seemed a very long time, although in reality it was probably only several seconds. I was very aware of my limbs shaking and, try as I would, I could not stop it.

I had just about got my emotions under control and was reaching for the ignition key to start the engine, when I saw it again.

It was on the side of the road, out of the main beam of the headlights which were glaring into the white fog dead ahead. The apparition rose slowly out of the mist, the disembodied face distorted in a silent scream, the arms rising again, pleading. I almost screamed myself, and jumped in my car seat with sufficient force to bang my head on the roof.

And then it was gone.

I stared hard at the spot, terrified. Every instinct told me to start the car and get the hell out of there. Then I saw it again, and all at once my mind started functioning again.

It was Mrs Long, of course, climbing out of the ditch at the side of the road. At some stage, she had fallen over into the mud, so that her back and part of one side were black from the peaty, clinging mud, and part of her front was white from the wet and torn nightdress. As she scrabbled and slid up the bank, turning with each desperate step, parts of her showed up in the half light, and parts merged, camouflaged into the night. The effect was heightened by the streaks and daubs of mud on her face and hair.

No wonder Billy and his girl had been so terrified.

I got out of the car and ran over to help her up. Grabbing the nearest hand, I pulled her upright and out of the ditch, and then held both her hands in mine. She stared at me, wild-eyed, completely insane with fright and shaking with cold.

Pulling the least muddy side toward me, I wrapped my arms round her in a great hug and shouted down her ear, as loud as I could, 'Mrs Long, what the hell are you doing out here at this time of night?'

She heard and understood me, despite the absence of

202

her hearing aid. She began shaking even more, and her breath came in great heaving sobs, but she did not reply.

'For God's sake, let's get you home before you catch your death of cold,' I shouted down her ear. She raised her head from my shoulder. The wildness had gone from her eyes and she knew who I was.

'Please,' she said, 'not home. They've come to get me, that's why I ran away.'

She was shivering uncontrollably, more cold now than fear. We were much nearer my house than hers, so it seemed the sensible thing to put her into the car and take her to the nearest warmth, and ring the police search parties from there.

I pointed to the car and ushered her towards it. She stopped at the door and said, 'But I'll make your seats all muddy.'

'Get in,' I said, and bundled her in, shutting the door firmly behind her. I drove home as fast as I dared through the mist, with the heater on full blast. She did not speak.

When we arrived home, my wife was in the kitchen. She had gone to bed, but, worried about my long absence, could not sleep and had got up to make tea. She met us at the door, took one look at Mrs Long and, in the manner of all women when faced with such a crisis, assumed full command.

She led Mrs Long by the hand to the bathroom.

'Make some fresh tea,' she said. 'That pot's cold, and bring it to us as soon as it's made.'

I did as I was told and put the kettle on. While waiting for it to boil, I rang the police and told them that I had found her, and what was going on. Peter answered it. There was a great deal of shouting in the background, so much that he could hardly hear what I said. The girl's father had got Billy by the verbal equivalent of the throat, and did not intend to let go.

'I'll come over to your house,' he said. 'The proceedings here are likely to go on all night, and I think the sergeant's enjoying it.'

I took the tea into the bathroom. Mrs Long had been washed like a baby under the shower, and was now clean

203

and powdered, and quite sane and rational, dressed in a pair of my woolly pyjamas and an old dressing-gown. Her own wet and muddy garment lay in a heap on the floor.

We drank the tea and waited for Peter, while Mrs Long told us all about the men in her attic, who had come to get her.

It was absolutely classic, straight out of the textbooks—senile paraphrenia. An old deaf lady, living on her own, who hears voices. The voices are very real to her, and often menacing. The instructions of the voices have to be obeyed. Mrs Long told us all about them. It explained everything. And now, because she had refused to obey them any longer, they were going to kill her.

When alone and hearing the voices, it is a state of actual schizophrenia, and by any criterion the old lady is certifiably mad; but contact with other people and reality soon dispels the state. To put her in the mental hospital would really be unnecessary as, within a few days, or even possibly hours, she would be sane again. What she needed was company, not hospitals, and a small dose of a psychotropic drug like largactil.

The mere fact of telling a sympathetic audience of the experience was rapidly bringing the whole episode into perspective. My wife slipped out and returned with a plate of cold beef sandwiches which the old lady ate ravenously, between several more cups of tea.

'I've been a silly old fool, haven't I?' she said. I nodded in agreement. 'I've imagined the whole thing, haven't I?' She paused for another swig of tea. 'Fancy me getting all worked up like that and frightening myself to death. I really did think that they were there, you know, and I really knew they were coming to get me.'

'You've been on your own too long,' I told her. 'You're all right now, but it will all come back if you are alone for too long again. I can give you some pills to help, but what you really need is company.

'I know,' she replied, 'but who wants to live with a deaf old fool like me? I can't pay anybody, you know.'

We were speaking to her in normal voices. She could not hear a word we said, but if we faced her directly and spoke slowly and distinctly, she lip-read every syllable.

The door bell rang. It was Peter, and we all assembled round the kitchen table and brewed yet another pot of tea. I explained to him all about the senile paraphrenia and said that I thought she would be safe to go home.

'Please, can I stay here?' she said. 'I know it's all in my imagination, but I know, if I go home, they will come back as soon as you've all gone.' She looked at my wife. 'Please. I promise not to be any trouble.'

We exchanged glances, and Ruth nodded her head.

'Is the spare bedrom ready?' I asked. 'If you go and get her into bed, I'll get an injection of largactil for her. Then we'll all have a good night's sleep.'

Mrs Long took her injection without a murmur; we said goodnight to the policeman and climbed thankfully between the sheets.

In the morning I took her a cup of tea, but she was fast asleep so I did not wake her. She was still asleep when I came home for lunch, and by tea-time, when she still had not woken, my wife was getting worried.

'Leave her alone till I get home from surgery,' I told her. 'I gave her a pretty good slug of largactil last night, and she was exhausted.'

She was still sleeping when I came back, so I went to rouse her. I had to shake her pretty forcefully before she stirred. Eventually she came to, but was still very sleepy and drugged. 'I don't like your injections,' she said. 'I'm not having any more of them.'

She sat up and shook her head.

'Ugh, I feel horrible.' Somewhat shakily, she swung her feet out of bed and stood up. 'Oh dear,' she said, suddenly remembering, 'I haven't got any clothes to get dressed in.'

'Never mind,' I told her. 'You go and have a shower, and then come and have some supper with us.'

She looked puzzled. 'That injection must have been worse than I thought, I could have sworn you said supper.'

'I did,' I said.

'Good Heavens! Have I been asleep here in your bed all day? I'm not having any more of your blasted injections.'

205

And she stomped off, somewhat erratically, to the bathroom.

Over supper we agreed that she could stay one more night, to sleep off the injection, as she put it, and I would take her home before surgery in the morning.

On the journey home she did not mention the men in her attic. I gave her a prescription for some largactil tablets and told her that I would ask Peter to get them for her.

'I'm not taking any of your pills,' she said. 'Your injection made me feel horrible.'

'Mrs Long,' I said, 'either you take those pills, or the men in your attic will come back, and next time I'll put you away in the nuthouse.' She knew I meant it, but it was still doubtful if she would take them.

During the course of the day I contacted everyone who I thought could help, who could call on her when passing—the social services, the district nurses and the police force. I almost rang the fire brigade as well, but thought better of it.

Peter was very good. He arranged to get as many of his colleagues as he could to use her house as a coffee shop, and the social services arranged for a home help to call twice a week.

For several weeks all was well. At least once a day, sometimes more often, a police patrol car was parked outside her house, and to my intense surprise she took her pills like a lamb. There was no more talk of men in her attic.

Once again my own visiting tended to become less frequent, and the home help rang up periodically for a fresh supply of pills. The police cars gradually became occasional instead of daily callers; even the home help, after some months, felt that she was no longer needed and was sent to work elsewhere.

* * *

The year slipped quietly by, autumn into winter; I had not noticed that there had been no recent requests for more pills for Mrs Long, and although I should have been, I was not aware that she had stopped taking them.

206

This oversight was brought home to me literally on Christmas Eve. Mac was doing the Christmas 'on call' and I was completely free. The family had gathered in force for the festivities and had been arriving all day. It was a miserable evening, wet and cold; the children had all been packed expectantly off to bed, and we were gathered round the fire filling their stockings, pleasantly mellow on Father-in-law's Christmas cheer.

The door bell rang. We were not expecting anybody, and off-duty time was so precious that any intrusion on it by patients was bitterly resented.

'Would you answer it?' I asked my wife. 'And if it's anything medical, tell them I've emigrated, or gone to church, or something.'

I picked up my glass and took a good swig. 'Better still, tell them the truth: I'm drunk, and you've had to put me to bed.'

She walked out of the room to the back door. All conversation stopped while we waited for her to come back. She was not long in returning. Poking her head round the door, she said to me, 'Can you come into the kitchen, please?'

I knew it was trouble without being told. I left the still-silent party and followed her out.

Mrs Long stood just inside the back door, absolutely soaked. She was wearing a coat but no hat, and her hair, plastered by the rain to her head, dripped on to her collar. Her hearing aid, hanging by its cord round her ear, hung uselessly by her face, also dripping water.

A pool of water was gathering round her feet, oozing out of her well-worn pink bedroom slippers, growing bigger with the drips from her coat as I watched.

Her eyes were wild and staring, not the complete madness of before, but rapidly heading that way. She carried a big old-fashioned handbag, and hanging half out of it, soaking wet, was her old white nightdress.

'Quick,' she said, 'quick. Draw the curtains, or they'll see me.' Dropping her bag, she grabbed at the curtain and gave it a hard yank.

Our kitchen curtains were primarily for decoration. The sink was under the window, and the view looked directly out over the lake. We never drew them as nobody could look in, unless they were coming to the door, and on the few occasions when we had closed them, they had trailed into the washing-up water.

The powerful tug from Mrs Long pulled them right off their runners, and as they swung away from the window they swept all my wife's cherished pot plants into the sink and onto the floor.

Mrs Long was not in the least contrite. 'Quick,' she said, 'give me some tea towels to put up. They mustn't know I'm here.'

I walked up to her, grabbed her by the shoulders and shook her. There was no point in shouting; without her hearing aid she would not hear, and she was far too pre-occupied to lip-read. I screwed her hearing aid back into her ear, water and all, chased the cord down inside her coat and produced the battery box. Turning up the volume as far as it would go, so that it produced that mind-splitting screech, I shouted into it as loud as I could, 'Mrs Long, what the hell are you doing here?'

It had the desired effect. It made her jump. My voice at that range and amplification was as powerful as those in her head.

I now had her attention.

'What the hell are you doing here?' I shouted into the amplifier again.

She took the earpiece out of her ear and shook it. I turned the volume down to cut off the screech. 'There's water in my hearing aid,' she said. 'It makes it uncomfortably loud. What did you say?' and she put the aid back in her ear and gave me her full attention. The wildness had left her eyes.

'What are you doing here?' I asked for the third time.

Quite calmly, quite rationally, she replied, 'I escaped. They came to kill me again. I only just got away in time.' She looked at the curtains, lying among the wreckage in the sink. 'Can we put those up as soon as possible, before they know that I'm here?'

She was as nutty as a fruit cake, and it was Christmas Eve, and she was in my house. To get her certified would be time-consuming and difficult; this was my precious day off duty and I had a house full of relatives having a party. And I'd still got the children's stockings to fill.

'Mrs Long,' I shouted at her, 'you've not been taking your damn' pills and you're getting hallucinations again. Those men are only in your mind. They don't exist. I warned you that I'd put you into hospital, and I'm going to have to do it on Christmas Eve.'

'Please don't put me in hospital tonight,' she said. 'I knew I'd be safe if I came to stay with you. I've brought my night things.' She bent down and produced the sodden garment from her bag. 'Oh dear, it's got all wet,' and she marched over to the stove, leaving a trail of water behind her, and carefully arranged it to dry over the hot plate.

'It'll soon dry there,' she announced. 'When it's dry, I'll go to bed. I won't be any trouble, and I've brought my pills.' She rummaged about in the bottom of her bag and produced the fruits of the last three prescriptions—three unopened bottles of largactil tablets.

The only trouble was that we had no spare bed. We had a full house, and the kids were doubled up with their cousins, all in a frenzy of pre-Christmas excitement. I did not want to spoil their Christmas with an old lady, terrified of bogy-men, wandering around the house when they were expecting Father Christmas.

The sensible thing was to ring the mental hospital and get her admitted, but at this time of a Christmas Eve they would not be keen, and she would have to be certified. The psychiatrist would have to come out and Mrs Long be carted off under protest, which would probably wake the children. Besides, it was a singularly uncharitable thing to do at this season of the year.

I spoke to my wife. 'Where the hell can we put her?'

'Well,' she said, after a moment's thought, 'she could go up in the attic, on one of the camp beds. What a Christmas, alone and certified mad in a mental institution.'

That decided it. She could stay, but it would have to be in the attic, and I suddenly remembered that the men out to get her were in *her* attic. I hoped to God they were not in mine, or if they were, that she would not hear them.

We took off her wet clothes and hung them up to dry. 'Please, don't give her any alcohol,' I told my wife, 'because I'm going to give her the biggest jab of largactil in the book, and they might clash.'

I went out to the car and took out of my bag several syringes and the box of largactil injections. I also brought in the largest ampoule I had of injectable glucose solution, used to restore diabetics from a low sugar coma. Walking up to the old lady and brandishing my largest syringe and the enormous ampoule, I told her, 'This is for you. One peep about any more nonsense and I'll give it you, all of it, and if you don't take your pills, you'll get it anyway.'

She said she'd take her pills, we gave her coffee and, when her nightdress was dry, took her up into the attic and put her to bed in the camp bed. I took four pills out of one of the bottles and watched over her while she swallowed them. Four was a pretty hefty dose and should put her out for the night. I waved the enormous syringe and glucose ampoule at her. 'Remember,' I said, 'one peep, and I'll give it you.'

'You won't need to do that,' she said, composing herself serenely for sleep. 'I'm quite safe from them here. Your attic is much too high for them to climb up and get me.' And with complete peace of mind she took out her hearing aid, closed her eyes and switched me off, together with all the other men who were bothering her.

The party had come to an end, the stockings were all filled, and I took the injections to bed with me, fully intending to give one to her if there was one sound from the attic.

In the event, there was not. After we left her she never moved. An army of excited children woke us very early in the morning, all eager to show us what Father Christmas had brought. I told them that Mrs Long was in the attic.

'Can we go and see her?' they shouted at once. 'Has she brought her pussy cats?'

'I'd better go and see if she's awake first,' I told them. She was awake, and completely sane. The largactil had done its job.

'Thank you for being so kind to a silly old woman,' she

said. 'I knew I'd be all right if I came here.'

The children swarmed into the room, carrying oranges, plastic toys, chocolates and a captured Harry cat. We left her, her bed a sea of wrapping paper and sticky sweets, with children and cat bouncing all over it.

Eventually they came down to breakfast, I stood over her while she took two more pills, and she appointed herself in charge of the washing up.

During the morning I went down to the island to feed the ducks. Mrs Long came with me. She was fascinated by them, and I had to tell her the origins and story behind every duck. As we were walking back she confided to me,

'You know, I feel safe here. They'll never get me here. I can still hear them, but I'm not listening to them and it's making them very angry. But it doesn't matter and I don't care.'

My Christmas spirits sagged. She would need another double dose of largactil at lunch time. Father-in-law had brought some of his very special wine. If she had that as well, she'd either go berserk or pass out cold at the table.

We went back into the house, she almost skipping with gaiety, and I a little apprehensive. I need not have worried: she was as good as gold. She helped prepare the vegetables, she washed saucepans—a real adopted grandmother.

The festivities went with a swing. I gave her extra pills, and behind my back she wheedled a glass of wine out of Father-in-law. Mercifully, all it did was make her sleepy, so that when the children went to bed she was happy to go with them. For luck, she had two more largactils.

The visiting relatives thought she was such a charming old lady.

My holiday was over on Boxing Day. It was Mac's turn to have a rest. He always insisted that I have Christmas Day off, because of the children, and then take over on Boxing Day. I thought that this was very generous of him, until I discovered that people must be *in extremis* before they would call a doctor on Christmas Day; hence, he was disturbed only very occasionally. Boxing Day, however, is just like any other, and it is fair game to disturb the doctor.

211

All the colds, chicken pox, indigestion and other miseries are carefully saved for Boxing Day, together with all the ailments that have been endured before Christmas and are suddenly bad enough to warrant instant attention.

The end result of all this was that Boxing Day was extremely busy and I hardly saw the family, let alone Mrs Long. Ruth was instructed to feed her the pills at frequent intervals, and Father-in-law was threatened with excommunication if he gave her any more booze.

During the course of the day, I had to call at the Church Army Home of Rest, where two of the elderly residents were quietly slipping away. In fact they had both done so on Christmas Day but, true to form, the good sisters in charge had not liked to disturb my Christmas and had left the formalities until today. I told them all about Mrs Long and, like the true angels of mercy that they were, they agreed to take her in the morning.

I made time the next morning to take her back to her house to pick up some clothes and, despite her protestations, deposited her with the Church Army, together with her three bottles of pills.

*   *   *

She stayed there exactly two weeks. The regular medication, combined with all the company and activity in the Home, was enough to restore her pretty smartly to complete normality. She pleaded with the sisters to let her go home and, as she was so active and well, we could not really stop her.

Once again I sought the aid of the social services and the police force, and once again her house became a branch of the police canteen, and the mental welfare officer called every week. As often as he was able, Peter made it his first task of the morning to light her fire and make sure she took her pills with the coffee. Whenever I was passing her house I called in, and on several occasions met Peter there and caught up on all the village gossip.

'You remember young Billy Wright?' he asked me one morning.

'Of course, I haven't seen or heard of him for ages,' I replied. 'What's happened to him?'

'They're letting him out today. You know he got three months for having intercourse with a minor, that girl that our good lady here frightened so much? Well, her father pressed charges, and he got three months for that, and they added another three months that had previously been suspended. I've got a bit of a problem. His parents have had enough and won't have him home, and the girl's fallen for him in a big way. She's been visiting him on every possible occasion and, by the way, she's six months pregnant and has fallen out with her father. She was down here last week and asked me if I could help persuade Billy's parents to take both of them in.'

'Are they going to?' I asked. Billy's father was a big tough tractor driver, as tough and as solid as his tractor and with about as much imagination. If he said no, he meant it, and not even an earthquake would shift him.

'That's the problem,' Peter said. 'I shall have to make certain suggestions that won't exactly please him, but I think he'll take them.'

I hated to think what those suggestions might be, for there was little that escaped the notice of our village policeman.

For one brief moment I thought of suggesting that they came as lodgers with Mrs Long, but just as rapidly dismissed it and said nothing.

She had been trying very hard to follow our conversation, but not really succeeding. 'What was that you said about a pregnant girl?' she asked.

Peter picked up her hearing aid and switched it on.

'Old dear,' he said into it, 'You've been listening to the light programme again. I keep telling you to tune into the home service.'

She smiled at him and smacked his hand. 'Come on,' she said, 'Tell me all about this girl.'

Peter began all over again and I left them to it. Whether the story he now told her had anything to do with the truth was unlikely, but no doubt it would be entertaining.

She seemed to be in good hands and, with the mental

welfare officer calling regularly, the whole situation was under control. I had not seen her for about a week when I came home for lunch one day, late, harassed and preoccupied with apparently insoluble problems.

Ruth met me at the door. 'Old Mrs Long's dead,' she said. 'The mental welfare officer rang a few minutes ago and wants you to go out and certify the death. I said you'd pop out before your lunch. He told me to tell you that he's informed the police, and the undertaker's men will be there when you arrive.'

This was a bit of a blow. Dotty she might have been, but not ill. There would certainly have to be a *post mortem*. I could not give a death certificate as I had not the remotest idea why she had died. The coroner would have to be informed. Still, I thought, if I went straight there, it would only take a few minutes, and the police could take over again.

All the way to her house I worried about whether she could have taken an overdose of pills; but then, I consoled myself, she had never given the slightest hint that she might do so.

When I arrived at the house, there was a solemn deputation waiting for me, undertaker's van and all.

'What happened?' I asked the mental welfare officer. Her front door was shut and a ladder reached up to her bedroom window. The window had been broken and they had obviously forced an entry.

He told me how he had called during the morning and found the doors all locked, the milk still on the step and all the curtains in the house still drawn. He had banged on all the doors and windows and, getting no reply, had gone off to fetch Peter. Together they had got a ladder and smashed the bedroom window to get in. Mrs Long was lying in her bed, and a big chest of drawers had been moved in front of the door to stop it opening—presumably to keep out the men from the attic.

'I've got a key to get in,' Peter said, 'but she'd put the bolts across, the first time she'd ever done that, so we couldn't use the door. It's my early shift, so I hadn't had a chance to call this morning.'

It sounds more like suicide than ever, I thought, as I went up the ladder and climbed in through the window. The room was still in darkness, so I opened the curtains, and looked round.

The chest of drawers was indeed wedged firmly against the door; it would have been impossible to open it from outside the room.

Mrs Long was lying in bed, looking very white and still. The first and simplest test of death is to raise an eyelid and look into the eye. In a dead person, the eye is glazed, fixed, and the pupil often dilated. The next step is to shine a light into the eye, to test for pupillary reaction which is absent in death, and finally to look into the eye with an ophthalmoscope and confirm by the characteristic appearance of the blood within the blood vessels. Last of all comes a check with the stethoscope that heart and breath sounds are absent.

Having taken my ophthalmoscope out of my bag, I raised one of her eyelids and looked into her eye. Mrs Long looked back at me.

'Hallo,' she said. 'What are you doing here?'

I gathered up my scattered wits and told her. She did not hear a word. 'Wait a minute,' she said. 'Can you see my hearing aid?'

It was on a chair beside her bed. I retrieved it, and she plugged in and adjusted it. 'That's better. Now tell me what you're doing here in the middle of the night.'

'It's not the middle of the night,' I told her, 'it's the middle of the day. I'd come to certify you dead.' And I told her what had happened, and about all the people waiting for me outside in the garden.

'Why are you still in bed?' I asked her. 'And why are you barricaded in? Are you hearing those voices again?'

Somewhat sheepishly, she admitted that 'they' had come again in the night, so she had put the furniture in front of the door to keep them out and taken a handful of pills to switch them off.

'They've gone again now, thank goodness,' she said. 'I had been a bit naughty, and not taken them,' pointing to the bottle of pills. 'Did I take too many?'

'I'll go downstairs, and tell all those people to go and get their lunch,' I said, and started to move the furniture out of the way. The chest of drawers was heavy—it was as much as I could do to shift it—and yet the old lady had moved it all by herself in the night.

Mrs Long got out of bed and wrapped herself in her old dressing-gown.

'If they're all going home to lunch,' she said, 'I expect that they'd like a glass of sherry before they go,' and she set off in front of me out of the room and down the stairs.

She opened the door and invited them in. Open-mouthed they entered. 'You are all expected to take sherry with the corpse,' I told them.

The mental welfare officer had two or three.

'Peter,' I said to him, as I manoeuvred him away from the others. 'This can't go on. If I insist she goes into an old folk's home, she'll discharge herself the next day, but she's got to have more company all day, someone actually living with her. Do you know of anybody who would be prepared to put up with her, in return for bed and board?'

He thought for a moment. 'Only young Billy and his girl,' he said, dismissing it as ridiculous, even as he said it. 'They're leading a dog's life where they are. Other than that, I can't think of anybody, but I'll bear it in mind.'

That afternoon Billy brought his girl to my antenatal clinic. She would have looked beautiful had she not been crying. I did all the routine checks and asked all the routine questions. Physically, everything was completely normal, but she was beyond being desperately unhappy, and Billy was as bad. They had no money and no home. He had lost his job, and they could not even afford to get married before the baby came.

The atmosphere in his father's house was vicious. The suggestions that Peter had made had not been kindly received.

'Can you not go back to your parents?' I asked her.

'He says he'll kill me,' Billy interrupted, 'and I know he means it.'

I told them all about my problems with Mrs Long, and how she was the old lady who had frightened them so ter-

216

ribly. If I could arrange it, I asked, would they be prepared to live with her, at least for a time, until I could convince her that she would be better off in a home?

It was the first ray of hope, and the first kind word that they had heard since his discharge from prison.

She answered for both of them. 'I've had so many insults in the past few months that insanity would be a nice change.'

'Leave it with me,' I said. 'I'll see what I can do, and let you know when I've done it.'

After evening surgery I went round to see Mrs Long. Peter was there up in her attic. I heard his voice as I went in.

'I tell you, there's nothing up here,' he was shouting.

'Have you been right up to the very far end?' she shouted back. 'That's where they hide when you're here.'

Peter emerged from the loft, covered in dust and cobwebs.

'For God's sake, Doc,' he said to me, and pointed at her hearing aid. 'Tell her to change channels; she's hearing those blasted advertisements on ITV again. Can't you get her to switch to the BBC?'

I told him about my conversation with Billy and his girl.

He turned to Mrs Long. 'We've had a stroke of luck. Doc's found a young man who will come and sleep here with you, and he'll keep those pests of yours out of the attic. I'll go and fetch him now. Oh, by the way, he'll have to bring his wife. She's pregnant, and he doesn't want to leave her alone.'

As quickly and as easily as that they were billeted on her.

'Get that spare bed made up,' he shouted at her, 'and when you've done that, make some coffee. I'll be back with them in half an hour.'

Mrs Long and I rummaged in innumerable cupboards and drawers before we found all the necessary sheets, blankets and pillows, and had just finished when Peter returned. The girl was crying, Billy looked pole-axed and was carrying their total worldly goods in one small suitcase.

217

In spite of being dotty, Mrs Long was no fool. She saw instantly that she was being used, and even more quickly that they needed help.

'Let's go and get that coffee,' she said, and led the girl by the hand into the kitchen. 'You can tell me all about it.'

Mrs Long and the girl took to each other in a big way. Billy was purely supernumerary and hung around, bashful and embarrassed.

Peter and I, like Arabs in the night, folded our tents and stole quietly away, wishing Billy the best of luck as we passed. The women never noticed our departure.

I called on my rounds the next day to see how they were getting on. A full-scale conference was in progress round the kitchen table, with the Vicar and the mental welfare officer.

Mrs Long rose from the table accusingly and wagged her finger at me.

'Did you know that these two weren't married?' she demanded. 'And her in that condition?'

'Well, yes, but . . .' I started, but she cut me short. 'You should have done something about it, and since nobody has, *I* am going to, starting right now.'

'Good,' I said and, pleading pressure of work, left them to it. Far better that she be obsessed with wedding arrangements than voices in her attic.

I heard later from Peter that it had all gone without a hitch. Quite a few people had turned up for the wedding, and most of them had got drunk in the pub afterwards. Mrs Long had been excused pills for the day so that she could enjoy it and, instead, Billy had performed a special exorcism ceremony in the attic, with good effect.

When she next came to the antenatal clinic, I asked the girl, now looking really radiant, how everything was going.

'Marvellous,' she said. 'Billy's got a job at last, and he likes it. Mrs Long won't let us pay any rent, but we buy all the food and she's knitting baby clothes like mad.'

'Is she still hearing voices?' I asked. 'Since you've been there, I've hardly had to see her at all.'

'She's very sweet, really,' she replied, 'and we make a

joke of the voices. I give her the pills every day, and Billy goes up into the loft every evening to send them away. She says that having someone to talk to about them makes them much less frightening, and if she does get scared, we talk about how much she frightened us that evening last summer, and then she's all right again.'

As I showed her to the door, I thanked her for solving my problem. She smiled, a really happy little smile.

'And thank you, too,' she said, 'for giving me a grand-mother. You know, I've never had one before. They're rather nice, aren't they?'

18

It was a perfect September morning, one of those mornings that, every so often, take me by surprise. The wide skies of Suffolk were wider than ever, reaching to the horizon in every direction.

Although mountain country is glorious, there is a sense of restriction in the valleys, a feeling that can only be overcome by climbing the mountain, to where the sky is free.

I had no need, that morning, to climb a mountain to feel the freedom all around me.

The sky itself was an all-enveloping picture. The red and yellow of early morning had gone, for the sun was just above the far trees, casting long shadows across the lawn. Where I had walked across it, I had left footprints in the dew that seemed to cast shadows of their own. The low-level light lit up every one of the myriads of spiders' webs in the grass, the beads of dew along their threads sparkling and flashing multicoloured dots as they awoke.

The few clouds were high and still and wispy. It was cold, a crisp, clean, frosty cold that promised to turn into a warm Indian Summer day as the sun rose into that empty, waiting sky.

I walked down the garden to the lake, to my favourite seat, an old fallen log by the food hoppers. Out of habit, the birds swam up as if expecting food, even though the hoppers were far from empty. Neither had I brought any with me, not even a few slices of bread. Perhaps they were just surprised to see me so early in the morning.

The telephone call that had got me up had been, to the caller, one of crisis and drama and imminent tragedy. Why people should perforate their duodenal ulcers at four o'clock in the morning, in the middle of an apparently good night's sleep, was a question that I had been unable to answer, either then or now; but perforate it he had, and was probably at this very moment having it repaired on the

220

operating table. I had sent both him and his nagging, worrying wife (the very probable cause of his ulcers) into hospital; he to have the operation, and she to accompany him, in the hope that the act of having to get dressed would stop her hysterics. It had not, but at least it had moved her out of my earshot. I had given him an injection of potent pain killer, and her a very large dose of tranquilliser.

After all the noise and excitement of her personal crisis and his pain, it was very peaceful just watching waterfowl on such a beautiful morning, and contemplating the mysteries of human nature in such a vast universe.

By now we had acquired a considerable collection of birds. The bulk job-lot we had bought from the bird garden still formed the backbone of the collection, together with the geese that had been payment for our first year's hard work. We had birds from every continent of the world: Maned Geese from Australia, Mandarins from China, Tree Ducks from Africa, and birds that circumnavigated the globe. It was always a great source of sadness to me that they had to be pinioned to stop them flying away and migrating uselessly into the middle of the Atlantic. There were pairs of birds here from more than fifty different species, and we hoped to breed from them all.

With a distinct sense of peace, I sat on the log, under that enormous sky, and watched the birds, newly attired in their winter mating colours, come to inspect me.

There is an old Japanese truth that, to appreciate anything, only one of it should be possessed. If there is only one rose bush in the garden, and this bush is only permitted to have one bloom, the anticipation of this bloom is intense pleasure. As it grows and unfolds, every petal is known and loved, and the perfection of the open flower truly appreciated. As it fades, the memory of that perfection will last until it blooms again.

If, however, the bush has two blooms, each one will only have half the attention it deserves, and a garden full of rose bushes will merit only a passing glance.

Any one of our pairs of ducks deserved the attention of a Japanese rose grower. Each was beautiful in its own way, but because of the sheer numbers and the diversity, none could get more, in this sense, than a passing glance.

The pleasure of their company, too, should have been incidental to their money-earning capacity, to enable us to pay the mortgage and buy their food, but it was not. The money-earning potential, for me at least, had become entirely secondary to the enjoyment their presence brought me.

I had to admit, as I sat on that log watching them, that I had become a collector. Whereas other people collect stamps or china, I collected ducks.

In the Japanese concept of things, the house was the rose bush, and the lake the rose. Every duck was a petal on the flower, a part of the whole.

Our house was like the rose bush in another, entirely English and practical sense: it was very susceptible to disease. The house had erupted into the fruiting phase of dry rot.

The tiny grey threads of the dry rot fungus had lain more or less dormant since Elizabethan times, eking out a very precarious existence down in the cellars. When the philistine had carted in all that mushroom manure, however, the fungus had seized on it like manna from heaven, and taken on a new lease of life. With its roots firmly anchored and fertilised, it had grown slowly, silently but inexorably throughout the compost, up through the brickwork to just about every window in the house.

The philistine had hastened its progress when he had put in the swimming pool, by blocking off the natural ventilation with green untreated wood set in wet cement. When it reached this green wood, the fungus spent a year or two thoroughly enjoying it, and then exploded out of it, fruiting spores like toadstools.

They grew out of the most unlikely places in thick clumps, long thin white stems capped with soft, soggy white heads. After a couple of days, the whole lot collapsed into a black, slimy mess. The first ones appeared through the sitting-room carpet, under the television set, and the second half-way up the window of the downstairs lavatory.

The Benny man had been summoned. In dismay he had walked round, poked his penknife into the wood and kicked clumps of the compost in the cellar.

'We can't cope with this, Doc,' he said eventually. 'It's too big a job for evening work, I'll have to get the Boss.'

The Boss came out that same night. Nobody ever called him anything else, either to his face or behind his back. Not very tall and now approaching sixty, he looked as if he had worked hard, and eaten well, all his life. Slowly and methodically, he went round the house. He was even more gloomy than Benny had been.

'See this here,' he said, down in the cellar, directly under the television set, as he poked his knife into the joists. 'Rotten. It's a wonder the floor hasn't collapsed on you before now.'

I watched his penknife flicking out great chunks of crumbling wood. 'What can we do about it?' I asked apprehensively.

'New floor, new windows,' he replied over his shoulder, as he walked along the wall, jabbing his knife deep into every beam as he passed, and leaving a trail of chippings behind him. 'Everything from here to the attics will have to be treated.'

Over coffee in the kitchen, he looked at me squarely.

'This has become urgent now,' he said in his matter-of-fact voice. 'I'll get everybody over here tomorrow, get all that rotten wood out and expose the brickwork, then we can see what we've got to do. All your walls will have to be treated, of course, as well as the wood.'

'How do you do that, paint it on?'

'Good God, no. Drill holes every few inches and inject it.'

I stared at him, visualising our house looking like a colander, with hypodermic syringes sticking out of it all over the place.

'Pressure job,' he added. 'We'll have to get the specialists in.' And as if to cheer me up, 'They give a twenty-year guarantee.'

He did not mention the expense, nor did he offer an estimate.

After he and Benny had gone, Ruth and I sat at the table, huddling miserably over the dirty cups. Once more our dreams of not being in debt had been shattered. For a few glorious weeks we had actually entertained that thought. Her maternal grandmother, a splendid old Lincolnshire lady, shaped like a cottage loaf and as deaf as a post, who ruled her family with a mixture of guile and brute force, had, having achieved her last ambition of outliving her sister-in-law, died peacefully on her eighty-fifth birthday. She had left us a small legacy; not a vast sum of money, but enough for Ruth to dream of new furniture, carpets and curtains, and me of ever more exotic ducks.

Now it looked as if it was all going to pay for putting the house back together, after it had been torn apart, and we had no idea whether it would be enough.

Still, as we agreed again and again, we had no choice, there was no other alternative.

True to his word, the Boss reappeared, at seven-thirty the next morning, with Benny and four other men. Naturally, we were not dressed. An army of wheelbarrows crossed and recrossed the kitchen as we tried to eat breakfast, carting out all two tons of that mushroom manure to a heap in the garden.

I escaped to work, dropping off the children at school on the way. On my return, at lunch time, our sitting-room carpet was in a heap on top of the manure and, as the Boss said, the problem was exposed. He was walking up and down the old greenhouse at the top of the garden, eyeing the metal poles that supported it.

'Come here,' he said peremptorily, as I approached, and marched off in the direction of the cellar. The old stone-flagged floor down there was shining wet from its recent scrubbing, and sprouting from it was an army of upright metal poles, all held up by hydraulic jacks.

'Look at this,' he ordered, pointing to the ends of the main beam, which had been sawn off about a foot from the wall. 'This wood's sound. We can save it.'

I looked up. The floor-boards had all been sawn off, too. A row of gaping holes in the wall, where the main timbers had rested, peered back at me. 'How?' I said stupidly.

'What is going to hold up the floor, when you take all those supports away?'

'Those metal poles in that old greenhouse. You're not using it and it's about to fall down.'

'No,' I said.

When I came home again, much later in the day, all the men had gone home. It was virtually impossible to walk in the cellar. Beside each jack was a metal pole, the lot growing like grass from the floor, their feet in plots of newly-wet cement and their heads screwed firmly to the joists above. Our greenhouse was a pile of shattered timber and broken glass on top of the mushroom manure.

Entirely unsupported at either sides or ends, our sitting-room floor floated free, on top of that sea of upright poles.

It had taken another three weeks for all the windows to be removed, replaced and treated, and I had been astounded at how much preserving fluid could be forced into the multitude of holes in the old bricks; but at last the job was done, and yesterday we had chosen a new carpet.

I rose slowly from my log, while the birds milled around unconcernedly.

'Ducks,' I said to them, 'next year, we expect great things of you. You've got to pay for that new carpet.'

Grandma's legacy had just paid Boss's bill but would not cover the new carpet. I ambled back up the lawn to the house and breakfast. The rising sun now left no shadows on the lawn and the dew had evaporated from all the spiders' webs. It was time to go back to work.

225